How to grow your dental membership plan

Marketing secrets behind my 1.4 million dollars of growth

Dr. Christopher Phelps DMD, CMCT

While the benefits of creating your own in-house savings plan are well demonstrated in this book, there may be limitations in your state which require you to register your practice and plan with your state's insurance commission. Seek the advice of a lawyer who is knowledgeable in this area to find out how an in-house savings plan is regulated in your state.

How to grow your dental membership plan:
Marketing secrets behind my 1.4 million dollars of growth

For information contact:
www.MembershipSavingsPlan.com

Book and Cover design by Soapbox Books

First Edition: October, 2016

Contents

Foreword

There are three elements of having ongoing substantial growth in a dental practice:

1) A steady stream of new patients,

2) Patient retention through an effective hygiene recare system,

3) Offering an in-office Dental $avings Plan.

When I think of unconventional, out-of-the-box dental marketing, marketing that truly comes from the heart, not the P&L spreadsheet, I think of my friend, Dr. Christopher Phelps from Charlotte, North Carolina. Dr. Chris knows more about attracting quality new patients than most of us in the profession. He is not afraid to step "out of the box" and create a new box. By coloring out of the lines he is able to creatively and effectively ease the financial pain of patients in need of ideal care; those who think they can't afford it. Chris's one, two, three punch has allowed him to grow his own practice exponentially. Now, through this book, he is helping massive numbers of dentists who may be struggling to gain the competitive advantage in their own hometown.

Chris believes in target marketing instead of the shotgun approach; being all things to all segments of the population. He instead uses what I like to think of as the rifle approach, knowing up front it is the 45-75 year old patients who live in active adult communities that want what he delivers; thus he delivers ideal dentistry to ideal consumers. These patients enjoy the finer things in life; looking good and feeling good is their mantra. The Wine and Cheese Receptions with an educational slant draw this group to his practice like moths to a fire. Each patient invited is asked to bring a friend, typically someone else in this age category. Chris believes in multiples, and word of mouth referrals are abundant in that look-good-feel-good patient base. By having an in-office Dental $avings Plan, patients without insurance find it very easy to access the dentistry they deserve.

If your practice is stagnant, it is not due to the economy or your competition. Sadly it's YOU! You too need to step out of the box. It will do you good to listen to Dr. Phelps' teachings so you too can achieve the practice of your dreams. You can have a practice with a large new patient base, a strong following of loyal patients who are happy to refer you to friends. Doubling your new patient number is as easy as 1, 2, 3. Keeping your patients excited and referring is a byproduct of following Dr. Chris Phelps' teachings.

Linda Miles,
Speaker, Consultant, Author, and Speaker Coach
lindamiles@cox.net
Virginia Beach, VA

Preface

If you have picked up this book, chances are good you and I are dentists cut from the same cloth. Let me take a guess at the type of doc you are (or strive to be). You're a go-getter. You want to be the best at what you do. You are not afraid to innovate, to improve upon the past. Dentists like us need to stick together. Our industry is changing and trends toward corporate takeover and cheaper-than-dirt dentistry are making it difficult for people like you and me to stay motivated. I see good doctors settle for mediocrity all too often. I see dental insurance having far too much control and my colleagues' clinical expertise ignored in favor of minimal restorative-based procedures. It is time we do something about this.

Carolinas Dental Center 2 Year Growth

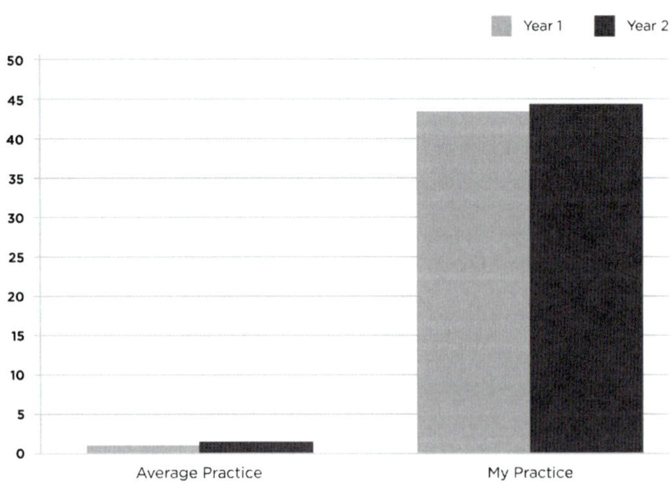

The good news: I am a firm believer private practice is not dead. In fact, while many private practices struggle to grow 1-2% a year, my practice has seen incredible growth: 43%, to the tune of $1.4 million over a two-year period.

How was this accomplished? I achieved such radical growth by tapping into dentistry's largest untouched market: fee-for-service patients.

My approach and my success are not isolated. I didn't get lucky. The process and the results are replicable. That means YOU can increase your revenue by 43%, if you have the drive and determination to follow my plan. If you are ready to take your future into your own hands, if you are willing to put some effort into your success, keep reading. I will share how to get more ideal patients and start growing your practice today.

PART I

THE BEGINNING

1

BREAKING FREE FROM THE BIG 3

It's no wonder doctors I talk to all over the world feel defeated. If you sit through happy hour at a Chicago Midwinter meeting or participate in any online forum, the underlying conversations always circle back to one of three tensions facing the private practice. I see them as weights dragging down the once-optimistic private practice dentist. I have worked hard to cut these tensions out of my life, and since then my focus, my resolve and my business have never been stronger.

Tensions Facing Private Practice

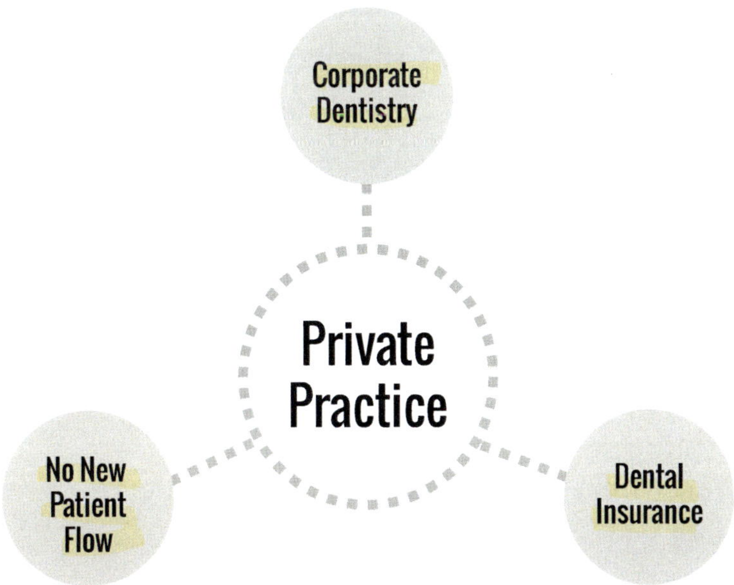

Tension 1: Corporate Dentistry

The thought of my profession being downgraded to the likes of strip mall haircut chains[i] makes me cringe. On the other hand, as a businessman and entrepreneur, I understand why many doctors choose to make their living within the perceived safety of the corporate model. It is risky to be on your own. You must be tenacious enough to go after what you want, but humble enough to learn from your mistakes. For me, freedom has always trumped comfort.

> *You can choose courage or you can choose comfort, but you cannot choose both. - Brene Brown*

For the sake of this book, I define "corporate" as any non-dentist-owned, non-dentist-managed dental practice. A place that has shareholders or stakeholders, that rely on a constant stream of profits as a return for their investment. These corporate-owned groups have money, huge buying power and leverage that can put the average dentist out on the streets. But, what they have in their rigid systems, they also lack in their flexibility. We have the adaptability and power to make swift changes, responsive in real time to our patients. So, if we are flexible and they are not, why do we hold so much fear? Why are we all so worried about the so-called corporate takeover?

For starters, the current climate does not favor entrepreneurship of young dentists. Lenders have significantly decreased the amount of money they are allowing new graduates to borrow because of their school debt, totaling upwards of $200,000-$400,000. So that takes purchasing a new or existing practice off the table. What's more, joining most private practices as an associate won't work out because many times these practices don't know how to attract enough new patients to support these doctors and allow them to make enough to cover their school loans. Many of these loans have interest rates in the 6-8% range, and this does not even factor in their basic living expenses. Couple these together and you can see why working for a corporate group can be enticing for the new grad and should lead them to less professional stress.

Think about it. The group takes care of supplies, HR, scheduling, marketing and often the retirement of its doctors. On the surface, it seems like a good deal.[ii] With more and more doctors getting closer to retirement age every day, fewer and fewer younger doctors are available to purchase their practices. This trend, toward the majority of the practices out there being corporately owned in the future, suddenly makes more sense.

Tensions Facing Private Practice [iii]

In a sample of 25 large corporate group practices, the number of dental offices went from 2,000 to 2,500 a 25% increase in just two years.

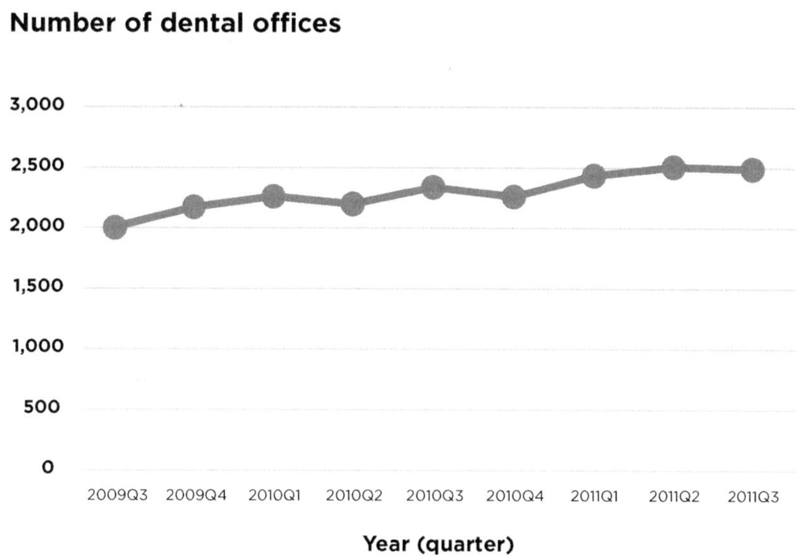

Compound the results from the graph above and I believe dentistry will look very different in 5-10 years. Not only are big-box dental groups burgeoning, private equity groups are jumping on the dental bandwagon. From Becker's Hospital Review on current trends in healthcare:

In the past decade alone, more than 25 private equity firms invested significantly in dental practice management, and some large companies in the sector have seen annual revenue of more than $100 million. This has evolved to the point where there are at least 10 large-scale dental practice management (DPM) companies[iv] actively growing.

Such investments are paying off for private equity firms: a Sageworks analysis found DPM investments generated the highest return on equity of the industries it examined.[v]

Corporate groups and those with private investors can afford to cater to high-cost patients and still stay in business, but as a doctor, if you go the route of corporate or private equity dentistry, you may as well leave your autonomy and ingenuity at the door.

All this adds up to scarcity and fear. The fear is that if a massive corporate group moves in down the street, your practice won't stand a chance. I used to think so too. But not anymore. Why? Because I know my market, and I know the patients I need in order to succeed today *and* survive tomorrow in the tough dental economy. I embraced the fear and found the courage to think outside the box for a new solution to this growing problem.

> *Fear can lead a man to wet his pants. Courage is what that man does with wet pants on. - Dan Sullivan, The Strategic Coach*

Tension 2: Dental Insurance

As dentists, we know dental insurance is nothing like medical insurance, but this understanding is an education our patients are still undergoing. Let me give you a few key talking points to help you help your patients who only accept treatments "that their insurance covers."

- Dental insurance is not actually insurance, but a dental benefit.
- Dental insurance, unlike medical, life or home insurance is not built on a model of a statistical unlikelihood a catastrophic event will occur. Dentistry needs to happen, and so dental insurance is meant to help offset regular costs, not cover large, unlikely costs.
- Because most people need dental care, caps are placed on benefits at $1,000–$2,000 per year.
- Dental insurance does not cover all necessary procedures/treatments patients may need.

We live the struggle. We want to help patients get better, but the antiquated model and misperceptions by patients of what dental insurance is supposed to accomplish ends up controlling our clinical ability to treat a patient's disease. Our patients end up doing the minimum, while we (practically) beg them to see the benefits of our comprehensive treatment plans.

Why does this struggle no longer control my approach? Because I see what most doctors don't. Sure, patients with insurance are frustrating, but they aren't who I want to treat. I want to treat the 114 million Americans without dental insurance. Keep reading and I'll tell you why.[vi]

Tension 3: Lack of New Patient Flow

When I was applying to dental school, I interviewed three dentists at different stages of their career. The first was near retirement, the second in his prime and the third was just beginning. I asked all three the same question: What did you like and dislike about dental school?

Shockingly, their answers were the same. They felt school adequately prepared them to treat patients well and provide excellent dental care, but all three lamented:

I have no idea how to run a business.

Now that I have been practicing for over a decade, I know exactly what these docs meant, and you probably do too. There is much more to dentistry than filling teeth. We need to know the ins and outs of hiring, leadership, marketing, turning our patients' needs into wants; the list goes on and on. The sad fact is we were not trained to be businesspeople. We were never taught how to make savvy financial decisions or do anything more than hang our sign on the front of our dental office and hope that patients would magically choose to come see us. While it is not our fault that we don't know what we weren't taught, it's up to us to figure it out. I have spent my entire career learning how to build a successful dental business, and how to make it thrive. I want to share my lessons so mistakes aren't repeated. My hope is that you and others like you will benefit from my experience as a result.

My greatest discovery has been a simple one. In order for our practices to grow, we need a steady stream of new patients. According to a survey done by the Levin Group, new patients account for approximately 40% of office revenue.[vii] We also know that on average, offices get 27 new patients per month.[viii] Does this sound like you? Did you also know the average office is losing 20 new patients per month? Patients move, pass away, find a new dentist for one reason or another, but ultimately they don't come back to see you. Ever wonder why your growth has stagnated over the years or gone negative despite what you thought was a healthy new patient flow? The reality is you have been blind to your patient attrition rate. If you gain 27 new patients this month, but 20 new patients from this time last year are not coming back in, you have actually only netted 7 new patients. Twenty of the 27 you received just replaced the production you did last year. Now hopefully, it makes more sense when I say if you can increase your new patient flow above and beyond your patient attrition rate, this will be your key to increasing your practices revenue. So, it makes sense to me that if I can increase new patient flow, I will increase revenue.

While this may not strike you as profound, that

realization was the catalyst that began my 43% growth spurt. As I was putting these pieces together, I was on the verge of changing the course of my practice for good.

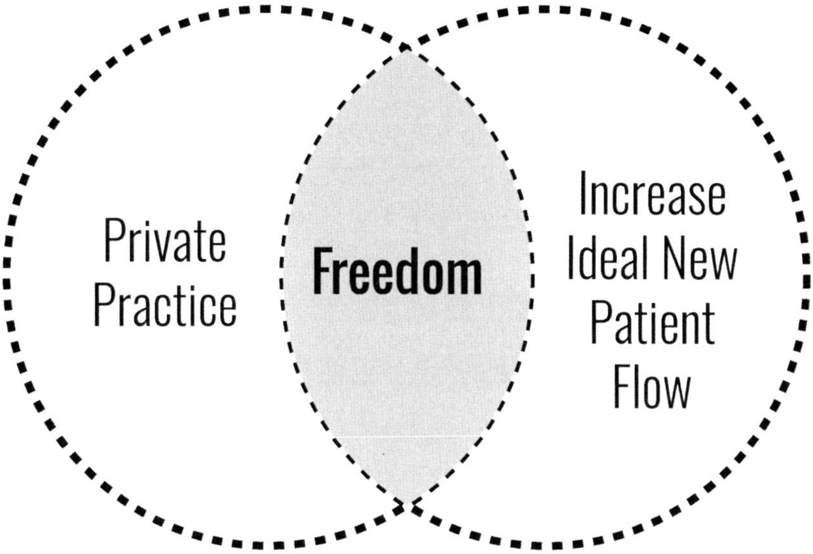

2

HOW TO MAKE THE MOST OF YOUR MARKETING

Half the money I spend on advertising is wasted; the trouble is I don't know which half. - John Wanamaker, Henry Ford (And just about any business owner I know)

How much do you spend on marketing your dental practice? An advertisement in a local paper can cost you several hundred dollars. A radio advertisement or billboard may run into the thousands over the course of a campaign. The marketers selling you the advertisements will justify the expense based on the number of people that you'll reach, but how many of those people are actually prospective patients? If you develop creative ways to target your marketing budget to a specific audience, you'll save money, increase your return on investment and give your practice the major growth spurt it needs!

Most big budget campaigns are like watering your lawn with a sprinkler. You use a lot of water, and the grass gets wet, but a lot of the water gets wasted on the sidewalk, the street, the mailbox and the weeds. A carefully targeted campaign is more like a soaker hose. You use exactly the amount of water you need, and you only water the plants you intend to water. There's almost no waste. A soaker hose is efficient and effective in ways that a sprinkler is not.

Many dentists gravitate toward 'sprinkler' campaigns because those don't take a lot of thought. You come up with a generic message, blast it at as many people as possible and hope you get an increase in business. As dentists, we're usually very exact. We don't fill every tooth in the mouth; we fill the one with a cavity. We don't take whole body x-rays; we look at the teeth and jaw. Yet somehow, when it comes to marketing, we lose our focus on the specific.

New patients are the lifeblood of any dental practice. According to a survey conducted by the ADA, more than a quarter of American dentists feel that they're not busy enough and want to increase the number of patients they see. If you want to run a profitable practice that can succeed today and survive tomorrow, you need to attract new patients.

In my own research, I've found that the average new patient is worth $1000 a year to a dental practice. Patients who need extensive work can bring your practice an additional $2500 a year. Marketing helps new patients find your practice, and data-driven marketing can help ensure that these new patients will be the best fit for you. Without data, you may be attracting a significant quantity of new patients, but most likely they won't be the sort of quality patients who keep coming back. You want patients who will value your practice, move forward with your treatment recommendations and refer friends, family neighbors and coworkers.

Using Data to Catch Big Fish

Many of my fellow dental practices follow what I like to call the "Hunting" method of marketing. They invest all of their marketing dollars in a single strategy, one that they often chose based on emotion or for the allure that a dental marketing company will do all the work for them.

This reminds me a lot of when I was growing up and my dad would take me deer hunting. I have many memories of getting woken up at the crack of dawn. Before the sun would even rise, I would be sitting in a deer stand. Sometimes we would spend as many as 8 hours a day sitting in the stand, hoping a deer would cross our path (also hoping that if it did, I was a good enough shot to hit it.). If you think about it, it was a significant investment of time and expense (deer stand, guns, camouflage outfits etc.). Why did we spend all the time, energy and resources hoping for one deer to cross our path and hoping our one shot was good enough to hit it? Isn't this how most of you do your marketing? Sinking a large investment into a direct mail piece hoping it will work, then having no idea why it didn't?

This reminds me of another time when my dad took me fishing. Normally when we would fish it was again a long investment of time, staring at the fishing pole and small floater that was bobbing above the water, hoping that one fish would bite. Then one time that we went fishing, something interesting happened. Almost immediately after I threw my fish hook and bait in the water, I immediately got a bite and reeled in a fish! It was record time! I couldn't believe it! I took the fish off the hook and put it in our storage container and re-baited the hook and BAM! Got another bite instantly! Crazy right? Then I got curious. I didn't put a worm on and just threw the hook in, and again, another bite! I looked over at my dad. He was experiencing the same thing; he couldn't catch the fish fast enough. So I got another idea. I remembered there being another pole in the truck. So I put down my pole and ran to the truck, grabbed the extra pole and threw both lines in the water. Sure enough, I got two bites at the same time! There I was, trying to reel in two fish and keep my balance. After this success, I got my dad an extra pole as well, and we were both pulling in fish two at a time. Hard to believe, right? It was the perfect illustration of how we should be doing our data-driven marketing.

Data-driven marketing is like fishing with multiple poles. You start out with small investments across a variety of media types: newspapers, radio, direct mailers, websites or community sponsorships. You track how many new patients each of your 'poles' attracts. If a certain pole doesn't get any bites, you stop fishing there, pull up stakes and drop your line in a different location. If you get a lot of bites in one place, you have two options. You can add bigger bait, meaning you can pump in more money to that campaign and see if it has an increased result. Or, if you can't add bigger bait, you can leave that pole in its place, drop another line in somewhere else and see if you can get some bites over there as well. You already use data and experimentation when you practice evidence-based dentistry. By applying that same scientific mindset to marketing, you can improve your results and increase your return on investment (ROI) from your marketing dollars.

Deciding Which Lures Work

A good fisherman knows that different types of bait attract different kinds of fish. He won't use the same lure for trout as he would for bass or for salmon as he would for catfish. Apply the same logic to marketing your practice. What sort of new patients do you want? In general, you want more of the sort of patients who already make your practice successful. If you specialize in pediatrics, you don't want to use marketing methods that attract adults without children at home. If your best patients are retirees, you probably shouldn't be trying to attract more young families to the practice. Focus on the patients who are the best match for your practice and your marketing dollars will yield a higher ROI.

Use data, not feelings, to determine who your best [illegible] are. Learn to run reports using your practice management software (or train a staff member to do it), and start asking questions. Who are the top 10–20 patients who have spent the most money in your practice over the last 12 months? What demographics do they share? What are they all reading? Where do they all live or congregate? Is there a pattern that connects them? Once you know the answers to these questions you'll have a better idea of where to find more patients just like them.

Once you know what kind of 'fish' you want, it's time to examine different kinds of 'bait.' For instance, if your best patients are young professionals, you may want to try to reach them through their phones, or along their commutes. If you seek retirees, AM radio ads and direct mail might be wise marketing experiments. If you'd like to connect more families with young children to your practice, you may want to focus your marketing on sponsoring Little League teams, handing out balloons at festivals or even visiting schools. Each of these styles of marketing is geared towards a particular type of patient. Little league teams won't introduce you to young professionals, and social media may have limited reach among older patients.

Check your intuitions about marketing ideas against data.

Consider surveying your current patients to find out which forms of media they consume. Read industry publications like Adweek[ix] to find out what different demographic groups prefer. Look at industry surveys. For instance, recent studies have found that Americans over 65 are most likely to watch television, read newspapers and listen to radio. And 95% of older Americans check the weather report daily.[x] So, if you're trying to reach retirees, you may want to schedule your ad spots around weather reports and buy ad space on the weather page of the newspaper.

So, now you've collected your data, analyzed it and learned how patients in your favorite demographics consume media. That means you're done, right? You can place ads and watch the new patients roll in. Not quite. Before you develop and place ads, you have one last job to do. You have to figure out what differentiates your practice from the 15-20 other dental marketing pieces your ideal patient is being exposed to every month. What makes you stand out?

Setting Yourself Apart With Brand Identity

To attract ideal new patients, you're going to have to show them what makes your practice special.

Brand identity is one of the basic principles of marketing.

Think of Coke. How do they advertise? They don't use slogans like: "We're Cola." "If you need a fizzy drink, choose us." "We're like every other soft drink on the market." If they did, who would choose their product? Why would anyone reach for a name-brand over an off-brand? Why would people keep returning to the same soda again and again, if the manufacturers and their customers were convinced that nothing set them apart from the competition?

When I've looked at dental marketing campaigns, it's clear that most of us haven't grasped the idea of brand identity. What's the most common marketing approach for dentists? A "$99 New Patient Special." If every dentist is using the same approach, how can patients find practices that best meet their needs?

If they can't tell the difference between dental offices, then they only have one other way to set us apart: by our price. Believe it or not, this $99 special is turning us into a commodity-based industry. In a commodity-based industry, the decisions of the consumer, in this case new patients, are based solely on price. Why? Because a .99 cheeseburger is a .99 cheeseburger, no matter where they buy it. Thus by the same logic, a crown is a crown is a crown. So with no other information to go from, they will always ask and go with the place with the cheaper crown, since price is the only way to tell us apart.

Think about this next time you launch a marketing campaign. I can tell you, if you choose to present your practice this way, the results get worse, not better. In my own market, the $99 special is now down to a $66 special.

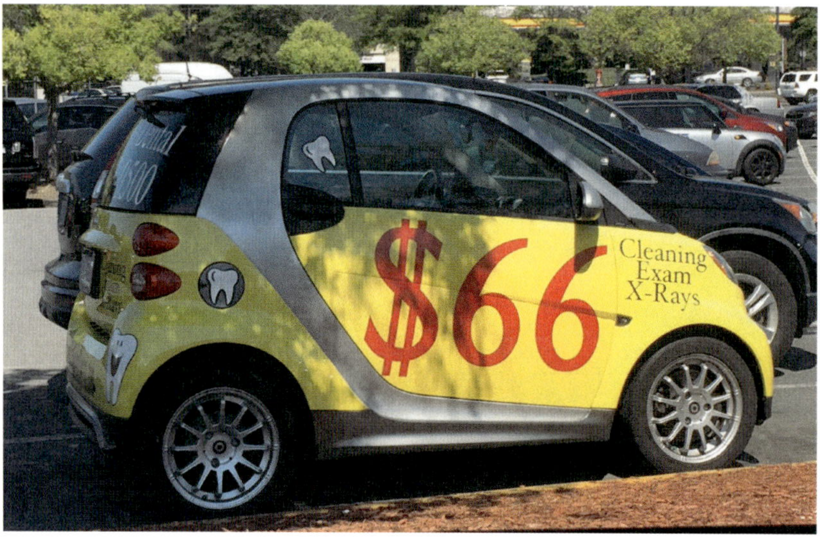

Photo taken at my local Walmart store

Before you know it, you will be just like the in-home cleaning services that have played the price game for so long, they now have to give away 1-2 hours of their service hoping to get their foot in the door, hoping you like their service, hoping you ask them back and hoping you pay them moving forward. Is this what you want for our practices?

Remember, the people responding to your ads probably haven't been to a dentist in a while. That means that you're targeting people who have been avoiding the dentist, possibly for years. To get them into the office, you need to show them how you can overcome the obstacles that have kept them out of the dental chair. Unless your ad has driven them to be price-conscious, a $99 special won't bring in the quality new patients your practice needs to thrive.

So, aside from price, what sets you apart? Why should someone come to your office? In my own practice, I created four services that set me apart and attracted new patients:

1. My offices are open outside of regular business hours. Many people can't leave work or school for dental appointments. Extended hours show that you're willing to meet them where they're at and remove this barrier for them. As a result I was able to make it possible for a larger number of patients to get in for an appointment and expand my client base.
2. I offer every level of dental sedation there is: laughing gas, oral conscious sedation, IV sedation as well as general anesthesia with our anesthesiologist that comes into the practice. I use the marketing message, "Forget you were ever here." Suddenly, I am attracting patients from 57 miles away. I am their option to get the large casework they need completed without the fear or memory of going to the dentist.
3. I offer multiple services at a single location. My patients get oral surgery, implant therapy for single missing teeth

to full edentulous arch treatments, orthodontia and routine dental care all in one office. This appeals to people who avoided the dentist because they were afraid that they had complex needs and would have to visit multiple providers to take care of them.

4. I realized, talking to my target market, how many of them would go to the dentist if they could just get to us. Transportation is a huge barrier for many seniors. I started sending Uber to pick them up and take them home. Barrier removed.

You have your own strengths. Take some time to identify them. For instance, a pediatric dentist might want to highlight the entertainment options available in his waiting rooms and examining area. If your office has peaceful, private bays, let prospective patients know. Do you take patients on time without long waits? Advertise your 'wait-free' appointments. If you have capacity, or open chair time to see new patients with dental issues today, tell them!

Listening to thousands of potential new patient phone calls captured by my CallTrackerROI phone service, I realized how many dentists have capacity issues. For most, if any patient, new or existing, calls your office today with a broken tooth, most cannot get them in for 3-5 days. Do you think they will actually wait that long? If this isn't you, and you have empty chairs galore, spread that message: "Can't get in to your dentist or any dentist? Call us today and we will see you today!"

Walk through your practice, and think about everything you do especially well. Go through past patient comments, and see what they've complimented. Make a list, summarize it with pithy statements, and make those specialties the focus of your marketing efforts. You'll see a larger return on your marketing campaigns and get more new patients who are likely to make your practice their permanent dental home.

While I had strong data and a steady stream of new patients, I knew I could do more. There had to be a way to overcome my existing patient attrition and increase my new patient flow to take my practice to the next level.

3
THE AH-HA MOMENT

My mom worked for AT&T for 32 years. When she retired I distinctly remember her telling me:

"Son, I am so glad you are going to be a dentist because guess what benefit they took from me first: dental insurance."

Ah-ha!

This was it.

My mom represents one of the largest untouched markets in the US: Baby Boomers, folks born between 1946-1964. If I could figure out how to get these patients through my doors, I knew it would change everything.

Baby Boomers are a huge segment of what many in our business call fee-for-service (FFS) patients. These are the 114 million Americans without dental insurance. Often we assume if they don't have insurance, they must not care about their dental health. Or, if they are FFS, they aren't financially capable of doing the dental work they need. While you think this may be the case, I would argue strongly it is a false presumption. You don't understand the mindset of this generation.

These fee-for-service retirees are anything but strapped for cash, and they highly value their oral health. You just need to understand the two main barriers keeping these patients from frequenting our practices now.

Baby Boomers: an Untouched Market

We have seen the trend. The US population is aging. In fact, between 2000 and 2010 the elderly grew at a much greater rate than the rest of the population: 15% vs. 10%. We are on trend to see people ages 65 and older go from 13% of the population to 19% by 2030.[xi] What is most interesting to me (beside the sheer number of Baby Boomers) is that, unlike my grandfather's generation, Baby Boomers share characteristics that make them perfect customers for the dental market.

Baby Boomers have money, and they are willing to spend it on improving their oral health, if you can overcome two obstacles for them. Consider these unique characteristics of Baby Boomers as consumers:

- Baby Boomers account for 70% of America's disposable income.
- Baby Boomers will inherit $13 trillion in the next two decades.[xii]
- Every year Boomers outspend the average consumer in nearly every category, from food, household furnishing, entertainment, personal care and gifts.[xiii]

• Baby Boomers spend over $150 billion dollars on trips annually. [xiv]

• Boomers account for 1/2 of all spending but are targeted by only 10% of marketing messages. [xv]

• Boomers are motivated by a 'bucket list' mentality, are health conscious and adventurous and want to stay youthful in appearance. [xvi]

Boomers are a huge opportunity for dentistry, so what is the problem? Well, it seems the Boomers themselves view dentistry as a cost they don't want to or can't incur. There is a belief that dentistry is too expensive without insurance. To folks like my mom, this thinking is a significant barrier to care. The ADA cites:

57 percent of those (Boomers) who have not visited a dentist in the past year cite lack of insurance and cost of care as the primary reason for not visiting a dentist. [xvii]

It makes sense, as most recently retired Americans spent their working lives with basic dental coverage, paid 100% by the company they worked for. They were used to paying zero dollars or a small, insignificant amount on a monthly basis, and as a result, their dental check-ups seemed to be 'free'. So the last thing they want to pay for is a dental insurance policy for them and their spouse. They can run up to $1200 per year. The barrier that is keeping them from our office is the thought that because they don't have dental insurance, they can't afford to see us unless they are in pain! To the logical person this makes no sense, because we as dentists know if they just came into the office for their routine checkup and cleanings, we can prevent them from having pain and other expensive issues. Regardless, it still doesn't overcome the barrier that they think because they don't have insurance, they can't come see us. Knowing this, what was I to do?

I knew what new patients I wanted to get through my doors, but I was faced with two issues:

1. How to put the retiree back in the driver's seat and remove the barrier of 'sticker shock'.
2. How to find and market to the group of Boomers I wanted to bring into my office.

4

BACK IN THE DRIVER'S SEAT WITH A DENTAL $AVINGS PLAN

I had been toying with the idea of offering an in-house dental membership plan, and with my newfound discovery of the obstacles keeping these patients from coming to see me, I began to think having my own Dental $avings Plan just might be the solution solution to both our problems. So what is an in-house savings plan? It is a way for fee-for-service patients to reap the benefits of dental care without the cost and hassle of dental insurance.

Typically an in-house plan covers basic procedures like cleanings, oral cancer screening and annual x-rays for a low monthly fee. It is much like joining Costco or Sam's Club. If you pay the monthly membership fee, you get a package of preventive care as well as discounted elective procedures. Here are the major benefits of offering an in-house dental membership plan:

- Complete control over price setting
- No third party paperwork
- No delay in patient approval for 'coverage'
- Attracts and helps retain new patients
- Breaks down the number one barrier to fee-for-service and

retired patients not seeing the dentist—no insurance
- Dental insurance companies have zero say in what procedures are 'approved' or not
- No annual caps
- No waiting for open enrollment
- Costs are predictable for patients
- Auto-renewal provides financial predictability for the office

The reason in-house dental savings plans have taken off, in my opinion, is the constant frustration dental professionals feel working with insurance companies. Normally a patient gets treatment and then you bill insurance. The insurance employs people who decide whether or not to reimburse you. They also employ the people who put my staff on hold when we call to protest a denial of claims. They employ marketers and lobbyists and advertisers to help them grow their business. There are even dental insurance companies in some states that are buying or building dental offices. Talk about a conflict of interest! So, even if an insurance company pays me $100, they know it is a procedure they should be paying me $200 or more for. So they will continue to pad their bottom line to deliver their shareholders the profits they demand.

Meanwhile, with a Dental $avings Plan, the patient joins the plan, I complete the procedure, and we're done. No billing them, since the service was included in their plan payments. No calls to insurance. I get paid, they get treatment, and everyone is happy. When you cut the insurance middleman out of the treatment process, you and your patients save money.

Additionally, when a patient signs up for a plan, they are much more likely to pay for additional services compared to a non-member. Consider Amazon Prime. In John Warrillow's book *The Automatic Customer: Creating a Subscription Business in Any Industry* he provides insight into the Amazon Prime effect. Prime members spend—on average—$1,224 while non-prime customers spend $505 per year. He calls the membership the "Trojan Horse." People who purchase from Amazon see the amazing value and convenience being a member provides and therefore seem to spend more. The membership also strengthens their loyalty to Amazon as a brand. Further, Robbie Schwietzer, vice president of Amazon Prime, tells Warrillow: "In all my years here, I don't remember anything that has been as successful at getting customers to shop in new product lines." To bring it back to dentistry; if I can get a new patient through my doors with the purchase of a plan, I now have a customer more likely to purchase needed treatment and ancillary products and procedures from my office alone. If they are a member here, why go anywhere else?

Also, plans are set up to auto-renew each month. This is an

incredibly important element of the plan for both the patient and the practice. Again Warrillow points out that a membership or a subscription model, "Increases the life- time value of a customer." Instead of selling a discounted exam to get someone through the door for $99 or less and never see them again, I have a customer worth $299 (at minimum) for the year, someone who has committed to come in and visit my office in order to "get their money's worth." Furthermore, since my patients are paying me the full $299 up front, there is no chasing people around and begging them to come in for their appointments. No-shows in your office will disappear because they have 'prepaid' for your preventive services.

It seems like a no-brainer. However, these plans have proven difficult for most dental offices to market well. The benefits are there, but they don't have enough people join to make them worth the trouble. Most dentists I know develop a plan or go with a group who provides in-house savings plan solutions, but they don't effectively market the plans to the right potential customers. It is a real struggle. If patients are already in office as an existing patient, they either have existing insurance coverage or already 'bought' into your value, and they are just fine paying your full fees. To many, being able to 'afford' your full fee is a status symbol or confidence builder, demonstrating where they are in life in their community. Now, if you try to 'talk them into' your dental savings plan, it may actually backfire; they will turn you down and be upset that you tried to 'push it' on them. This doesn't mean you ignore educating them and alerting them that you are offering the plan, it just means you should let them know: "Many other patients, such as yourself, have chosen to save some money off the care they need and choose to purchase it." You ultimately leave the decision to purchase or not up to them. Again, this is for the Baby Boomer, the fee-for-service patient, who is not already coming to see you, not your existing patients.

Fee-for-service patients make up a smattering across demographics. Single-parent households or small business employees might be good targets, but most dentists I know are stuck in a marketing rut and aren't effectively marketing in-house plans or regular services well. Marketing is a large aspect of practicing dentistry; yet again, as my dentist friends told me way back before starting school, it was not taught, so we as a profession struggle to know if our marketing is working. Before I could start to think about my in-house dental savings marketing, I had some work to do.

5
PUTTING THE PIECES TOGETHER

Whenever I am developing a new marketing campaign, I focus on the 3 M's: Market, Message and Medium. In my experience, all three need to align in order to see a campaign work. The reason so many dental offices don't see more new patients is the lack of congruence between these three things. They may have a target market identified, like working professionals, and a message that works—*"We are open after work!"*—but the medium through which their message is being conveyed misses the mark. Perhaps they are sending post cards that are being tossed in the trash. If they had done just a little research, they would have found that working professionals say they feel they are missing out if they are not on Facebook or Twitter every day,[xviii] so perhaps a sponsored Facebook ad would be a better medium.

Defining Your Market

Who is your ideal patient? Can you list the characteristics? If you haven't ever mapped your ideal patient profile, now is a good time to start. Here is a short list of things to determine about the ideal patient for your practice: [xix]

- Demographics
- Characteristics
- Purchasing and shopping behavior
- Fascination triggers

First, make a list of your ideal patient's demographics. This includes things like average age, income level, area of residence and gender. Perhaps your ideal patients are:

- Female
- Over the age of 55
- Live within a 10 mile radius of the office
- Middle to upper class

Then, list defining characteristics of this ideal patient, things like hobbies, activities, values, profession, likes and dislikes. Your ideal patient may have these characteristics:

- Values health and looks
- Active
- Retired or works part time
- Values social interaction
- Avoids traffic and late-night events

Then, do some research to see how your demographic prefers to shop. Are they online? Do they read the local paper? Are they at the movie theatre every Tuesday and

Thursday evening? Honing in on buying behavior will pay off dividends.

Finally, one of the most interesting ways to define your ideal patient is to be aware of their fascination triggers. These triggers are written about by Sally Hogshead in her book: *Fascinate: Your 7 Triggers to Persuasion and Captivation.*[xx] In her book she explains which triggers motivate people. The seven are: prestige, trust, lust, power, alarm, mystique and vice. According to Hogshead if you are able to speak to your ideal customer's fascination trigger in your marketing, you will better attract your ideal patient.

What is Your Message?

Once you have an ideal patient profile, you can craft your message. If you know you are speaking to an active, retired female who values her health and has a strong prestige trigger, your message may be something like:

Don't let your unwillingness to show your smile hold you back from living your best life ~ Come see Dr. Smith for a free cosmetic consultation in our spa-like office.

Treat yourself to the best smile of your life, you deserve it!

Once you know who you are speaking to, it is much

easier to tailor the language to fit the persona.

Finding the Right Medium

Finally, you want to make sure you are getting your well-tailored message to the right people through the right medium. If you want to attract active, 55+ females, you may not want to spend all your marketing dollars on sponsoring a t-ball team. A better medium may be advertising during a popular show on public radio or a print ad in the lifestyle section of the local paper. Find out where your ideal patients are, and go to them.

If your market, message or medium do not align with one another, you will be wasting valuable time and resources missing the target.

Lightning Strikes

As I was going through this process for my in-house dental membership plan and thinking about the Baby Boomer opportunity, lightning struck.

I was seeing a patient who mentioned to me she had recently moved into an independent-living retirement community a short ten minute drive from my practice. She said it was a wonderful place to live, as everyone there was over 55, active and completely independent. She mentioned this particular community had over 3,500 homes.

Boom!

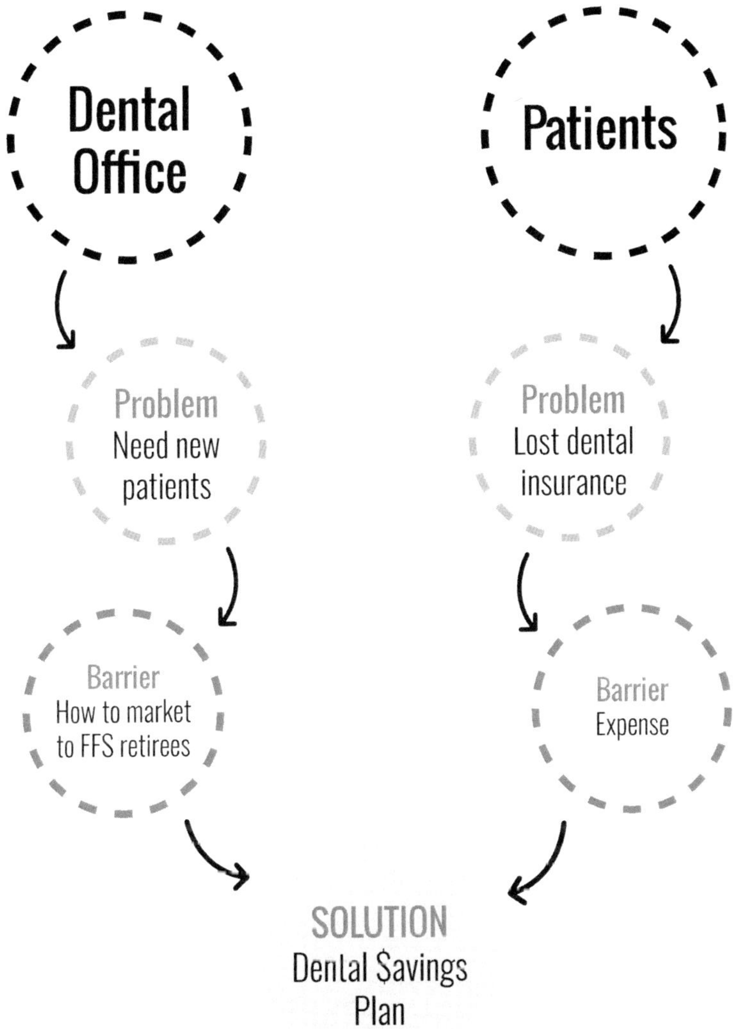

Just like that, I had honed in on my market: a group of retired Baby Boomers in a central location. My patient went on to explain they had a community-based magazine that was distributed regularly. So there was my perfect medium.

I was able to pay for a full-page color advertisement for $900. To my surprise, as a magazine sponsor I was also offered the opportunity to come on-site to offer an educational seminar. I knew that my message had to be a home run if I were to successfully attract my market to this event; it took some time, but once I figured it out, it completely changed the course of my practice.

PART II

GROWING MY DENTAL $AVINGS PLAN AND MY PRACTICE WITH WINE AND CHEESE

6
CHEERS TO TAKING A CHANCE

One thing I knew about Baby Boomers is they like one-on-one interaction. They are the generation of handshakes, and while they are tech savvy, an in-person interaction could help build trust and show transparency[xxi] (two things Boomers demand from brands). Boomers don't like to be treated as if they are elderly. These folks have bucket lists a mile long and want to live life to the fullest. I knew I couldn't just show up with a dull PowerPoint presentation; I had to make it fun and exciting.

At the time, my wife and I were novice wine connoisseurs. We had just returned from our first trip out to Napa Valley California. It was wine country and we loved it! We loved the educational element, learning the science behind the wine-making process. We were awestruck by how there can be over 500 wineries in the same geographical location and still be differentiated enough from one another to be unique and attention-grabbing. That first trip out, I will admit, I let the wine tasting experience get the best of me. I inadvertently joined the wine club of 10 of the 12 wineries we visited. Many of you know the old adage: "What happens in Vegas stays in Vegas." What I didn't know was, "What happens in Napa follows you home every month!" I swear, every month boxes and boxes of wine kept showing up at my house, thanks to all of the memberships I had joined. I realized quickly I had to do something with all the wine.

Thinking about how much I enjoyed the Napa wine-tasting experience and how I had an upcoming educational seminar, I asked myself: "If I valued this wine-tasting experience, would the people in this community, many of whom can't physically travel to Napa themselves, appreciate it if I brought Napa to them?" Thus, the lightning of inspiration struck and my message was born: "If you can't get to Napa Valley, I'll bring Napa to you! Join me for an educational seminar on the top five issues facing the aging population and enjoy some of Napa's finest wines and cheese with me."

Historically, Boomers have been major wine consumers, and while Millennials have caught up to them, they are still the second-largest wine-drinking demographic:[xxii]

Total Wine Drinking Population by Generation

(Percentage by generation)

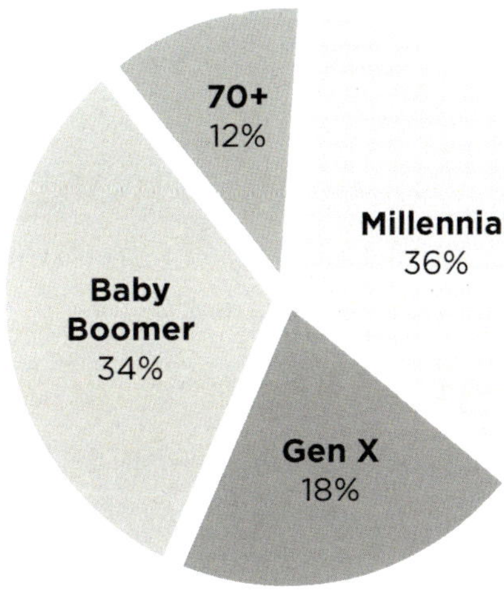

The First Wine and Cheese Event

So there I was, about to start my first presentation. The tables were set with brochures about our practice, business cards and pens with our logo and website and phone number on them. I brought about 8 bottles of wine from my newly formed collection along with a fruit and cheese plate one of my team members picked up before the event. As I didn't know what kind of wine they would enjoy, I brought two bottles each of Cabernet Sauvignon, Pinot Noir, Chardonnay and Sauvignon Blanc. The stage was set; two of my team members, my Dental Assistant and my Treatment Plan/Financial Coordinator were with me and ready to serve. I had no idea if anyone would even come; to my surprise, 60 people showed! It was a great turnout. Like most times when I speak to a new crowd, I had my Financial Coordinator introduce me. I was wearing a business suit and tie, so I looked professional. After I told the crowd a little about our dental practice, I turned my attention back to them and asked them three questions that would ultimately be a game-changer for my practice and life.

Here I was, talking to my market. It was too good an opportunity not to ask questions about them and their dental experiences to date. I started by asking them for feedback, telling them there would be no judgement from me toward their answers. I just wanted to know the truth. So I asked the following:

1. How many of you have been to the dentist within the last year?

From that question 10 of the 60 people in the room raised their hands. In my head I thought: "Geeze, that isn't good!"

2. How many of you have dental insurance?

Surprisingly, the same 10 people raised their hands. I thought to myself: "Interesting, I may be on to something here."

3. How many of you would have gone to the dentist if you had dental insurance?

To my surprise, the 50 people who had not been in the last year, all raised their hands. In that moment it hit me. There is a barrier that is keeping the overwhelming majority of these great patients from coming into our practices. This was an obstacle I had no idea existed. I then started thinking back to my mom's situation and put the pieces together. The source of this problem lies in the mindset of the person who is retired. When they were working, they had an abundance mindset. Abundance, as Dan Sullivan would describe it, means resources are unlimited. If I am generating income every month and spend too much money this month then I will be okay, because next month I will spend less to compensate. When Boomers saved their entire working life for retirement and then that monthly income is gone, they switched to a scarcity mindset. This means resources are not unlimited anymore. Every month, the money they saved is getting less and less and less, and their only hope is to have enough money to make it to the end. As a result, they are very protective of their funds, and everything seen as an expense. Since their company probably paid for their dental insurance, they had no idea how expensive it can be. Their coverage was the first thing they lost when they retired; their thoughts then became: "I'm on a fixed budget now, so I can't afford dental insurance." As a result of this thought process, their next mindset was: "Well, if I don't have dental insurance, then I can't go to the dentist unless I'm in pain." We all know that if they just came in for their preventive appointments, they would avoid such problems and expense down the road. So even though this line of thinking does not make any sense to us as dentists, this is the root cause keeping these amazing people from becoming our patients.

After the presentation was over, I spent a few days processing this revelation. Now that I had identified a real problem, I set to work creating a solution. My theory was that if I can just get them over this obstacle and get them into the practice, and if we do find a problem, they would probably move forward with treatment that day. I asked myself: "What can I offer them, similar to dental insurance, so they would be motivated to come into the office, but which is more customized and provides more benefits?" I needed my own in-house discount membership plan, which I would end up calling my Dental $avings Plan. With the solution to the problem in hand, the only thing left to do was to create my own plan, while trying to make it as simple for my team and these patients to understand as possible.

7
CREATING THE DENTAL $AVINGS PLAN

While I knew there were turnkey options out there, I wanted to make sure my product would be perfect for my specific market. Before designing my Dental $avings Plan, I asked myself the following questions.

1. How much are retirees paying for dental insurance now, and can I beat it?
2. What services come with traditional insurance?
3. Can I offer the same services for less and still make money?
4. Can a $avings Plan be a win-win for my office and my patients?
5. What financial impacts can a Dental $avings Plan have on my bottom line? Is it worth it?

Out of these five questions, my Dental $avings Plan was born.

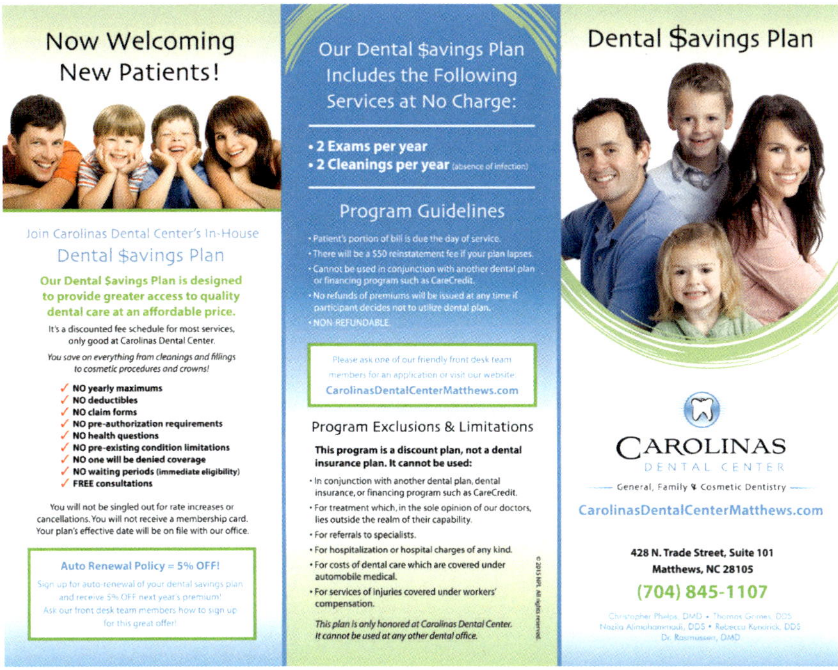
Now Welcoming New Patients!
Join Carolinas Dental Center's In-House
Dental $avings Plan
Our Dental $avings Plan is designed to provide greater access to quality dental care at an affordable price.
It's a discounted fee schedule for most services, only good at Carolinas Dental Center.
You save on everything from cleanings and fillings to cosmetic procedures and crowns!
✓ NO yearly maximums
✓ NO deductibles
✓ NO claim forms
✓ NO pre-authorization requirements
✓ NO health questions
✓ NO pre-existing condition limitations
✓ NO one will be denied coverage
✓ NO waiting periods (immediate eligibility)
✓ FREE consultations
You will not be singled out for rate increases or cancellations. You will not receive a membership card. Your plan's effective date will be on file with our office.
Auto Renewal Policy = 5% OFF!
Sign up for auto-renewal of your dental savings plan and receive 5% OFF next year's premium! Ask our front desk team members how to sign up for this great offer!
Our Dental $avings Plan Includes the Following Services at No Charge:
• 2 Exams per year
• 2 Cleanings per year (absence of infection)
Program Guidelines
• Patient's portion of bill is due the day of service.
• There will be a $50 reinstatement fee if your plan lapses.
• Cannot be used in conjunction with another dental plan or financing program such as CareCredit.
• No refunds of premiums will be issued at any time if participant decides not to utilize dental plan.
• NON-REFUNDABLE.
Please ask one of our friendly front desk team members for an application or visit our website:
CarolinasDentalCenterMatthews.com
Program Exclusions & Limitations
This program is a discount plan, not a dental insurance plan. It cannot be used:
• In conjunction with another dental plan, dental insurance, or financing program such as CareCredit.
• For treatment which, in the sole opinion of our doctors, lies outside the realm of their capability.
• For referrals to specialists.
• For hospitalization or hospital charges of any kind.
• For costs of dental care which are covered under automobile medical.
• For services of injuries covered under workers' compensation.
This plan is only honored at Carolinas Dental Center. It cannot be used at any other dental office.
© 2015 NPI. All rights reserved.
Dental $avings Plan
CAROLINAS
DENTAL CENTER
General, Family & Cosmetic Dentistry
CarolinasDentalCenterMatthews.com
428 N. Trade Street, Suite 101
Matthews, NC 28105
(704) 845-1107

Front page of my Dental $avings Plan brochure

Truth be told, I had no idea how much retirees paid for dental insurance. So, I did a little digging.

AARP[xxiii] is one of the largest dental insurance providers to seniors, so I went there first. I simply looked up rates in my zip code. Annual payments for my area were between $520 and $767. With those plans, seniors received discounts on: exams, cleanings, x-rays, fillings, root canals, gum treatment, extractions, denture repair and crowns.

Dental Plan(s)

Quote for **2** dental plan(s) for **1 person(s)** living in **NC 28173** starting **08/01/2016**.

Compare	Plan Name	Type	Deductible	Maximum	Premium	Next Step
	PPO Plan B	**PPO**	**$100**	**$1,000 Per Person**	**Monthly Cost:** **$43.32** Coverage starts: 8/01/2016	Enroll Save Quote Plan Details Find a Dentist
	PPO Plan A	**PPO**	**$50, waived on Diagnostic and Preventive**	**$1,500 Per Person**	**Monthly Cost:** **$63.93** Coverage starts: 8/01/2016	Enroll Save Quote Plan Details Find a Dentist
Compare						

Pro Plan B

Summary | Deductibles | Maximums | Diagnostic (exams, x-rays) | Preventive (cleanings) | More links ▾

Deductible per calendar year per person:	$100
Maximum per calendar year per person:	$1,100
	You pay
Office visit:	20%
Exams:	20%, 3 per Calendar Year
X-rays:	20%
Cleanings:	20%, 3 per Calendar Year
Fillings:	20%
Root canals:	50%
Gum treatment:	50%
Extractions:	50%
Denture repair:	50%
Crowns:	50%
Orthodontics:	Not a covered benefit

If a dental insurance policy was in the range of $520-$767, the average for my area would be around $600. To me, that seemed expensive; no wonder so many retirees weren't interested in being insured! For my office, I knew I needed to be able to cover my costs, while also overcoming the sticker-shock keeping retirees from coming to the dentist. Before I priced my savings plan, I raised my regular fees about 7%. This had been in the works, as it had been 3 years since I had increased any fees. As a result, I would now be able to offer any D$P member a discount off all the procedures and services we offered (a win for the patient) but without crippling my bottom line (a win for me). After doing the math, factoring in my overhead, I determined I could offer my D$P for $299, half what it would cost them to get dental insurance.

Dental $avings Plan

BENEFIT PREMIUMS

Plan:	Total Annual Cost:
Single	$299 (savings of $250 off our normal fees)
Dual*	$575 (savings of $575 off our normal fees)
Family** (3)	$752 (savings of $720 off our normal fees)
Family** (4)	$917 (savings of $1295 off our normal fees)
Each additional	$110

Diagnostic and X-rays

Service	Coverage
Comprehensive Exam (new patient / initial visit)	100%
1 Annual Exam (children under 18 = 2 per year)	100%
1 Emergency Exam (problem focused, 1 per year)	100%
4 Bitewing X-rays (1 time per year)	100%
Periapical, First Film	100%
Periapical, Each Additional Film	100%
Complete Series X-rays or Panorex (1 every 5 years)	50%
CT (3D imaging) scans	50%

Preventative

Service	Coverage
Child Prophylaxis (2 cleanings per year)	100%
Adult Prophylaxis (2 cleanings per year)	100%
Fluoride (2 per year, no age limit)	100%
Oral Cancer Screenings (2 per year)	100%
Additional cleanings per year	20%
Dental Sealants	20%

This price point does a few things. I can promote it as 50% less than the average cost of insurance (which is a huge selling point), and also provide other services at a 10%-15% discount to members who purchase the $299 plan.

Compare Out-of-Pocket Fees

Plan Premium, Product or Service	Dental $avings Plan Membership	Carolinas Dental Center's Regular Prices	Average Dental Insurance/AARP Costs
Annual Premium (single)	$299	$549	$480
Annual Premium (family of 4)	$917	$2,212	$1,492
Deductible	$0	$0	$50
Cleaning & Exam (twice per year)	$0	$260	$0
Lumineers/Veneers	$1,212	$1,347	$1,600 (not covered by most plans)
Dental Implants	$1,843 (You're saving $205!)	$2,048	$2,000 (not covered by most plans)

Save over $1,400 compared to Average Dental Insurance/AARP in the first year!

For my particular plan, I decided to include discounts. I offered a 10% discount for major procedures, such as crowns, implants, dentures and root canal therapy. I also offered a 15% discount for minor procedures, such as fillings, periodontal treatment like scaling and root planing, CBCT's, tooth whitening etc. These percentages can vary depending on your office margins. The important thing to remember is that because this generation is expense minded, the discount satisfies their desire to get a little something off for doing what they need to do.

Remember, you are now going to have a patient in your chair that is ready to move forward with your treatment recommendations. Without these discounts, your chair would still be empty. Let's put it another way using a crown fee of $1200. Would you rather collect $1080 ($1200 + 10% discount) toward that crown you are now doing, or would you rather collect 100% of $0, because you are not doing the crown at all? You can guess which one I decided to choose.

Our basic plan for $299 will include:

- ✓ **1 Comprehensive Exam**
- ✓ **1 Annual Exam**
- ✓ **1 Emergency Exam** (used any time during the year)
- ✓ **2 Cleanings** (non-Periodontal based)
- ✓ **2 Oral Cancer Screenings**
- ✓ **2 Fluoride Tooth Desensitizing Treatments**
- ✓ **4 Bitewing X-rays**
- ✓ **Any Individual X-rays needed throughout the year**
- ✓ **50% OFF Panorex or Full Mouth Series of X-rays and CT (3D imaging) scans**
- ✓ **20% OFF Additional Cleanings, Dental Sealants, Fillings, Core Buildups, Oral Surgery, Root Canals**
- ✓ **15% OFF Crowns, Veneers, Periodontics, Dentures, Partials, Implants**
- ✓ **$1,000 OFF Invisalign**
- ✓ **$325 Teeth Whitening**

To demonstrate their attraction to this discount, I remember being up at the front desk when a potential new patient walked through the front door. He did not have an appointment, but he had heard a lot about our Dental $avings Plan from someone in his neighborhood. So he asked me: "So, this savings plan of yours, if I buy it, I can get 10% off a crown?" I told him "Yes!" He then asked: "Well, what if I have five crowns that need to be done? Would I save 10% off all five?" To which I replied: "Yes, of course!" He got so excited he bought the Dental $avings Plan right then and there and made an appointment with us to examine him, and if we agreed with the diagnosis, complete those five crowns that day. He then did something I did not anticipate. He used his cell phone to call another dental office across the street from us, technically closer to his neighborhood, and canceled his appointment with them. Apparently he was scheduled to get his five crowns done that day at that office. But, after talking to one of his neighbors who had our Dental $avings Plan, he wanted to get his work done with us instead. I felt bad for the other dental office and their lost production, but that is the difference maker for this market; it benefits those that offer a D$P.

Interestingly, people join the plan for more reasons than the low premium. Some come for the amazing price point of the preventive services, but others are drawn to the discount on Invisalign® or veneers. For us, this is

nt, as we are able to offer them all of the preventive
to keep their teeth healthy during teeth straightening or veneer prep. It is a win-win for everyone.

Join Carolinas Dental Center's In-House
Dental $avings Plan

Our Dental $avings Plan is designed to provide greater access to quality dental care at an affordable price.

It's a discounted fee schedule for most services, only good at Carolinas Dental Center.

You save on everything from cleanings and fillings to cosmetic procedures and crowns!

- ✓ **NO yearly maximums**
- ✓ **NO deductibles**
- ✓ **NO claim forms**
- ✓ **NO pre-authorization requirements**
- ✓ **NO health questions**
- ✓ **NO pre-existing condition limitations**
- ✓ **NO one will be denied coverage**
- ✓ **NO waiting periods (immediate eligibility)**
- ✓ **FREE consultations**

Of course the greatest thing about offering an in-house plan is the control my associates and I have over treatment planning. Patients also feel a great sense of freedom over their own oral health.

8

9 KEY LESSONS LEARNED

Since its inception, there has been a lot of trial and error involved in refining and perfecting my Dental $avings Plan. One of the reasons this book exists is to help others avoid mistakes I've made, as well as those of others who have tried to implement their own membership plan. If you get nothing else from me, make sure you consider the following key lessons learned. It will save you time, energy, frustration and money.

Key 1: Don't overcharge for the service

I have watched far too many doctors overcharge for their in-house savings plan. They price the plans a fraction less than the AARP price and can't sell them to the Boomer market. It makes sense, because there is not enough of a contrast between their savings plan and the AARP price. Remember these folks are savvy shoppers who want to get a good deal. If the margins don't work with your current regular prices, perhaps raising your base fees can help. In my experience a price point of $499 will not sell.

Key 2: Keep your price point attractive, but not at a cost to you

In one of my offices, the $299 was not enough to cover the two hours of hygiene time per year and the dental exam. So, I had to get creative. I let my associates know if they would be willing to waive the $15 I would pay them to perform their exams, then I could give them an unlimited opportunity to present treatment to a Baby Boomer (remember these folks have money and value their health). They agreed, and because of it, they each collected an average of $1254 per patient in other services over the course of the year.

Key 3: Choose your stance when combining deals

In my office, we offer third party financing, such as Care Credit, to help folks get the treatment they need but at a monthly expense their budget can handle. Many times these companies seem to take what looks like a huge percentage of the case to allow us to offer an interest-free financing option. Yes, it can equate to 10-14% of your case fee, but many of you also know that without it there is no treatment acceptance and thus no case to be done. If possible, you can offer patients longer terms for their financing, which would then lessen your costs for most large cases, say $5000 or more. But, there should still be enough of a margin to make it work for both you and the patient, especially if they can't get all the treatment done without the financing option. For example, when I do my implant and hybrid denture cases, a procedure I teach other general dentists to do at the Phelps Institute, I'm charging $18,000 for the case. Let's do the math. My cost for six implants, the final custom-milled titanium bar I have fabricated and the final tooth set up and processing to create the completed restoration is $2140. Let's say the patient chooses to finance this over 12-24 months interest-free and use their 10% D$P discount. My cost to do this is around $4320 total. So with the $18,000 case fee and you take out the $2140 hard fee and the financing fee of $4320, I am still left with $11,450 for a procedure that takes about four total hours of my time to complete. That means I am collecting $2885 per hour of my time (the average dentist collects $500 per hour). At $2885 per hour, it makes sense to let the patients finance with Care Credit and let them use the 10% D$P discount as well, especially if this is the only way the case could be completed in the first place. Ultimately, I encourage you to do the math on your procedures and choose your stance; see which cases it makes sense for and which it doesn't for you. If you don't allow them to combine the D$P discount with the financing option, here is the language you use when explaining why to your patient:

"What is more valuable to you, Mrs. Jones, getting the discount and paying 10-15% less today or spreading the full amount over time? The choice is yours."

This takes me to the next key.

Key 4: Stand firm on the $299 up-front payment

When it comes to them paying the $299 for the Dental $avings Plan, I recommend your patient pays the fee all up front. I do not allow my patients to break this payment up over time. One reason is that I feel if they are not able to afford the $299 up front, then they are probably not a right fit for my practice, nor will they be able to afford any treatment needed. In addition, if you have added up my full fee for everything they receive in their first preventive visit with us, they would have spent $347. So, for my plan at $299, they are still getting a great deal.

Key 5: How to handle the Perio patient

We all know the struggle of the perio patient who does not understand the difference between a prophy and scaling and root planing. Since the D$P offers two cleanings per year as part of the package, how do we handle that patient who needs scaling and root planing? Think about it this way; once a patient receives their scaling and root planing, what do we call their cleaning moving forward? Perio maintenance. How many times a year, ideally, should they be receiving this Perio maintenance to control their disease? It's recommended four times a year. For this patient, I recommend you educate them on their periodontal disease and explain why this is not a prophy and consider the scaling and root planing they need as a minor procedure. Then, let them have a 15% discount on all the quadrants they need performed. You will educate them on what perio maintenance is and why they need four per year. My fee for this procedure is around $150 per visit, which is about $600 per year in total expense. As a plan member, I allow them to use their two "cleanings" for two of the four perio maintenance appointments they need. So I will only charge them $300 for the year for the two visits not covered by the D$P, while still offering them the 15% minor procedure discount off that rate.

Key 6: Establish an auto-renew system

One of the greatest lessons I learned was to create a system to automatically renew their plans after 12 calendar months. This saves my team an incredible amount of time. They don't have to track patients down and discuss renewal; they simply charge the patient's card when their 12 month cycle ends. It has also allowed for a 90% retention rate over two years in my practice. It is convenient for us and for the patient.

Key 7: Beware of in-network insurance conflicts

If you are an in-network provider, make sure to check the agreement you signed with that insurance company to see if you agreed to offer your in-network patients the lowest fee. So, if you have already agreed to charge these patients 20-40% less than cash-paying patients, you need to ensure the discount you provide Dental $avings Plan members does not take them below the price points you set for your insurance patient. Major procedures should be fairly easy to manage; however, the comprehensive preventive treatments for $299 may be an issue.

A few things you can do:

1. Discount your fees for the insurance patient so it matches the D$P member fee.
2. Raise the D$P fee to match the insurance member fee.
3. Split the difference.
4. Figure out a way to get out of the insurance game altogether.

Key 8: Commit to grassroots advertising

Fear of public speaking is listed as one of the top fears humans have. For many of you, the thought of getting up to speak in front of a large group of potential patients can be unnerving. This is why you would much rather send out mailers or let the radio transmit your message for you. Unfortunately, if there is one thing I have learned, it's that the only way to reach this group of fee-for-service patients is to meet with them. They are skeptics. They want to be able to look in your eyes and know they can trust you. They need to shake your hand. They are a group that values their own time and therefore sees the value in you taking your time to meet them.

Key 9: Set realistic expectations

You will grow your practice with an in-house membership plan. You will increase your new patient flow. You do have the ability, as I did, to make millions doing it. However, it does not happen in a day. Keep your expectations realistic and keep at it; don't let any little hurdle or obstacle or SNAFU stop you. Whatever you are facing, there is always a way around the problem. Remember, with every frustration, there is a breakthrough ready to occur.

"Always focus on the front windshield and not the rearview mirror." - Colin Powell

9
THE SECOND WINE AND CHEESE EVENT

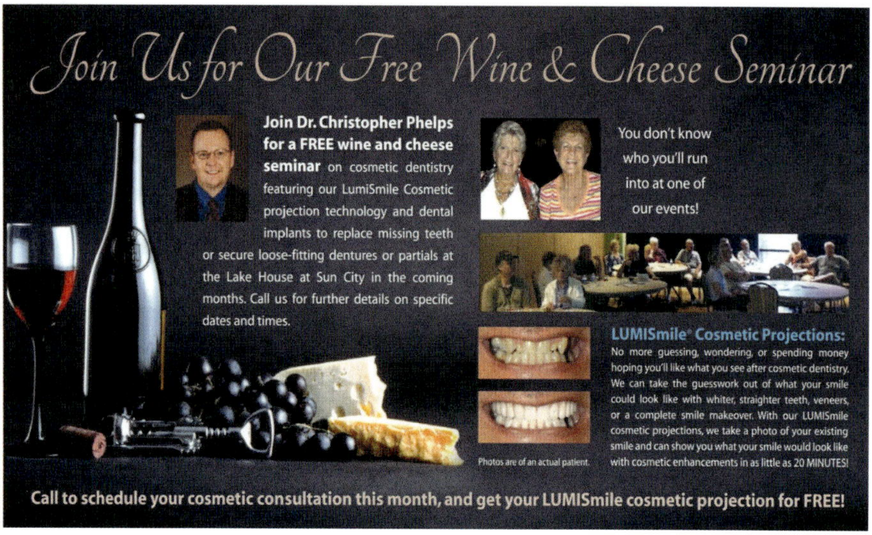

I hosted our second wine and cheese event about a month after our first. Having uncovered the reason we are not seeing more of these retirees in our practice, I was now ready to unveil our Dental $avings Plan as the solution.

For the second event, we connected to the Activities Director of the retirement facility. They assisted us in reserving a space and managing a sign up system. Residents could RSVP for the event at the center, and the Activities Director could relay the information to us so we were prepared with enough Dental $avings Plan brochures, application pages and similar materials about our practice, (and of course plenty of wine and cheese). In anticipation of the success I knew our Dental $avings Plan would have, I had created a Square account for my iPad, so we could charge their credit cards the $299 there on site. In addition, we were using a software application called LogMeIn, so we could have access to our schedule at the office and make everyone an appointment that night. The time for the presentation was at hand, and sure enough, we had another 60 people in attendance!

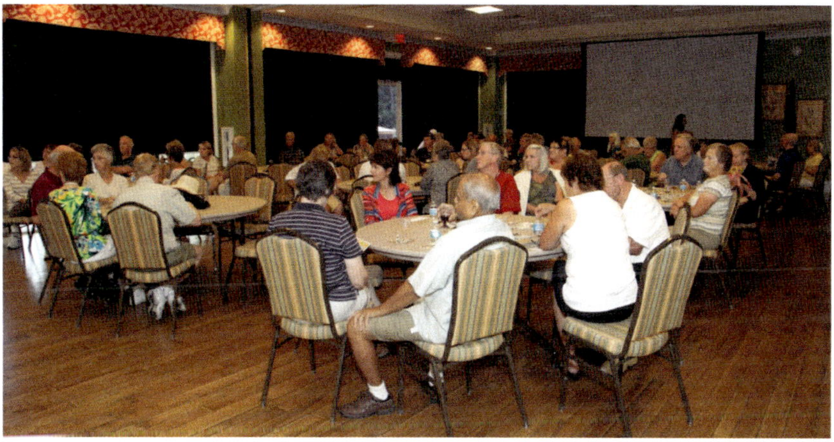

Attendees of the second wine and cheese event

I was prepared. I selected a variety of wine from my collection to take along: reds, whites, rosés and blends. I had my presentation together; full of interesting information about oral health as you age. I had an amazing assortment of cheeses and fruit to pair with the wine, and I had a support team there to help pour and sign people up for the plan on the spot.

I felt I had done everything right. My team confirmed my suspicion and said I connected to the group; they said the audience was engaged throughout the presentation and really seemed to trust me. I had made the presentation more educational on the whole, with the only promotional piece coming at the beginning as I presented the Dental $avings Plan. I asked the same three questions I had asked the first presentation, and sure enough, got the same results. 50 of the 60 people in attendance didn't have dental insurance, nor had they been to see the dentist in the past year. Sounds like success, right? The problem was this: my team said I knocked it out of the park, so surely all 50 bought the Dental $avings Plan or at least made an appointment to come to the office right? Wrong! Turns out we did not sell one Dental $avings Plan that night, nor did we make any appointments. I was baffled and disappointed. I thought I had failed. And thought to myself: "Was this a total waste of time? Had I been completely wrong about it all?"

I went over the night in my mind again and again. But it still didn't make sense. Many of you may have thrown in the towel at this point; after a few days of analyzing the event, I decided my instincts couldn't be wrong. I needed to press on and continue doing the events. Then, an amazing thing happened. Over the course of the next month, 45 of the 50 attendees without dental insurance either called and scheduled appointments or came to the office for an appointment and purchased the Dental $avings Plan. In addition, all ten of the attendees with insurance made appointments as well. Success!

In hindsight, it makes more sense to me now why they didn't sign up right then and there. Remember in Key #8 when I described this generation as skeptics? They really do have a mentality of: "Okay, sounds great, but what's the catch?" or "Sounds too good to be true." No wonder they didn't buy at the event! They had to take the Dental $avings Plan brochure and application page home and study it in detail, most likely looking for 'the catch'. When they couldn't find one, those 45 early adopters made the commitment to try us out and thus change the course of my practice forever.

How to treat the "First 45"

Our first handful of Dental $avings Plan buyers were treated like royalty. Not that every patient we see isn't, but these folks were exceedingly important. Why? Well, they were the first to use the plan, the first to talk about their experience to others and the first to let us know where we were falling short. Their experience and feedback was invaluable to the success of the program.

Remember, these retirement communities are like small towns. Everyone knows everything about everybody. They all talk. Over time the experience of the first 45 was relayed to others in the community. As a result, after each wine and cheese event, we got more and more patients. Another interesting phenomenon that took place as word in the community was spreading about us, and our trust factor was increasing, 50% of those without dental insurance were paying for the plan at the events, while the other 50% made appointments and would sign up for the plan when they were in our office. I would even have four to five people show up at the very end of the presentation, grab a glass of wine and say, "Sign me up for this D$P thing we keep hearing so much about!"

10
THE FINANCIAL IMPACT

Warrillow highlights another interesting point in his book about the true value of a subscriber: they buy more. Remember the Amazon Prime example? Turns out, once you have a customer who comes to you for a product (in our case, it is the preventive services offered with their Dental $avings Plan), they are more apt to purchase adjunct products. A story in *Businessweek* highlighted the enormous potential impact the subscription mindset has on add-on purchases from the article:

> ...customers spent as much as 150% more at Amazon after they became Prime members. Subscribers not only ordered more often, but after paying the $79 fee, they started buying things at Amazon that they probably wouldn't have in the past. Since shipping was always speedy and free, members saved themselves a trip to the store for things like batteries and coffee beans. "In all my years here, I don't remember anything that has been as successful at getting customers to shop in new product lines," Robbie Schwietzer, vice president of Amazon Prime, told Businessweek.[xxiv]

This exact phenomenon occurred in my office as well. Because these patients had already purchased the $299 plan, a few interesting things happened. First, they were more open to moving forward with other treatment I suggested, and second, they asked for, and purchased, elective procedures. I am 100% certain that if they had not already been sitting in my chair, they would have never come to me for these accessory services. What does this look like in terms of money? In two years I sold 957 plans at $299:

957 x $299 = $286,143

Each of the 957 patients on average has gone on to spend an additional $1254.

$1254 x 957 = $1,200,078

Total revenue: $1,486,821.00

If we want to look at cost, there is of course a cost to hosting these events. I spend, on average, $130 per event. That is the cost of the wine and the snacks. I also pay for the time of two of my team members to be there for two hours. So, say I have done 20 events a year; my costs have been around $2,600 x 2 = $5,200. While they didn't teach us much about business in dental school, I've learned enough since then to know that the 1.4 million in revenue is well worth the $5,200 investment.

The Added Value of Referrals

My office has several internal systems for guiding patients to say 'yes'. I am a certified Cialdini trainer and have found the Principles of Persuasion invaluable to my practice. The specific principle we use with our Dental $avings Plan members, once they are in office and are happy with our services, is Reciprocity. You see, they have access to hundreds of fee-for-service patients just like them when they return to their community. We can get in front of a limited number with our wine and cheese events, but harnessing the power of their referral leads to exponential potential for the office.

How to use the Power of Reciprocity for Referrals

Once your patients are through your doors, you have the opportunity to ask them to refer your office to friends. Where I see many doctors make mistakes here is not that they don't ask, but that they ask in the wrong way. For example, how many times have you tried: *refer x people and get free whitening?* I hear consultants tell their dentists to run such giveaways to drive new patients to their practice all the time. So what is wrong with enticing people with a gift such as this to get them through the door or motivate them to refer folks to your office? The problem is this: it isn't a *gift.* It is a *reward.*

If you make an appointment or referral, ***then*** you get whitening. The whitening only comes after an action or behavior by the patient—it is a reward for them doing something we want. A gift, on the other hand, is given without expectation of getting anything in return. Why split hairs? One reason is local law. In Oregon [xxv] for example, you cannot reward patients for making referrals without facing legal trouble. Secondly, most dentists don't know rewards, as opposed to gifts, have very little influence over patient behavior. Research from Dr. Robert Cialdini [xxvi] and his team shows that gifts have more influence over a patient than rewards. Think of it this way: a new patient schedules and is rewarded with whitening. What is their motivation to come to your office after they have received their reward?

On the other hand, if you gave them a gift first, how might it change the outcome? Let's say after that initial exam you said: "We are so glad you chose our office; here are a few gift options from us; why don't you choose one you'd like?" You see, having a choice of gifts is important because the gift itself is important. Not only should it be unexpected, but it should also have some value and significance for that person. Without this, the gift has no real influence power, so ultimately it's just an expense for you. Imagine if I gave you a nice stainless steel coffee mug, something that could keep your coffee hot all day long; if you drink coffee you might value this gift but if you don't drink coffee, what did I just give you? An inconvenience. Now you are staring at it wondering: "Great, what am I going to do with this, use it as a paperweight?" To avoid this, we need to have a couple potential gifts and let the patient choose the gift that has value to them. When you have truly engaged the Reciprocity Principle to the fullest, and the patient acknowledges that gift and says "thank you", then you can say: "My pleasure! Oh, and if you happen to know of anyone looking for a good dentist, will you tell them about us?"

A Dental $avings Plan is so much more than 'just another program'.

A Dental $avings Plan can increase:

- New ideal patient flow
- Treatment plan acceptance
- Referrals
- Elective procedures
- Practice revenue
- Community awareness

On the flip side, a D$P can decrease:

- Stress
- Open chair time

We all hate it when we start our clinical day, and by 9am

the Hygiene schedule from 10am to 3pm has already fallen apart, due to same-day cancellations. What is your team to do? Normally, we would look ahead in the schedule to see if anyone can come in sooner. The problem you run into, however, is that because the majority of people in your practice have dental insurance, they have to wait exactly six months and one day for their recare visit with you, otherwise their insurance company won't pay! Well, if the majority of your patients are retirees who have your Dental $avings Plan and they don't have any time restrictions, now you have an option. You could call one who is booked out three weeks and ask if they wouldn't mind moving it to today. Because they are retired and their schedule is flexible, many will come in and fill that cancellation. If they are due to renew their plan, you may even get some collections for filling that spot. Now you have 2-3 weeks to fill the open chair with a new patient who may call in. Do you see the potential here?

PART III

GROWING YOUR DENTAL MEMBERSHIP PLAN

11
FINDING THE RIGHT MARKET

Baby Boomers as a market, wine and cheese events as a medium and the Dental $avings Plan as a message has been a homerun for my office. I truly believe anyone can see the same success using this formula. However, I realize proximity to such high concentration of Baby Boomers may be a challenge for some doctors. In this section I will reveal all my secrets for how to pull off a successful wine and cheese event, and also offer some alternatives for those who are unable to locate an active retired community.

HOW TO FIND YOUR RETIREE MARKET

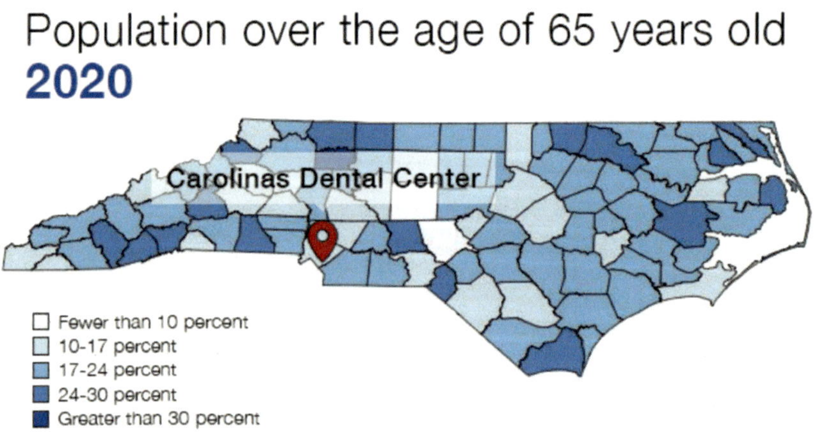

xxvii

We all know Baby Boomers can be found in all reac the nation. However, they may or may not be nicel centrated in these active independent communities. Rule number one, don't assume because you don't see these communities, they don't exist. Remember, I had zero clue there was one near me. Do some research. There are countless online resources for folks looking for retirement communities. Here are just a few:

Retirement Living Information Center
Website: www.RetirementLiving.com
Cost: One-time fee of 24.95
Resource: Retirement Community Directory among other resources.

America's Top 100 Best Master-Planned Communities
Website: www.RetireNet.com/top100
Cost: Free access
Resource: Search top 100 communities by state.

A Place For Mom
Website: www.APlaceForMom.com
Cost: Free, but you must create a profile to access information
Resource: Locate senior living communities by zip code.

Alternative market: SBM's

If the retiree market does not make sense to you, small businesses are another great market.

If you talk to business owners around town, they'll tell you about the soaring cost of health insurance, costly compliance with federal and state regulations, and how their costs keep rising. Meanwhile, they're afraid to raise prices, because they can't afford to lose customers.

It all adds up to another year without raises for their loyal employees. At a time when Walmart, McDonalds and other big companies are offering higher wages, how can small businesses compete? Most owners are afraid that they won't be able to keep their most competent staff members for long.

I'm sure you're wondering what all of this has to do with Dental $avings Plans. If someone isn't getting a raise this year, why would he be interested in a new Dental $avings Plan?

A Dental Savings Plan is a way to grow your practice by providing value to local small- and medium-sized businesses (SMBs). So SMBs are in a fix: they can't really afford to offer raises, but they need to offer something in order to retain employees. Health insurance is getting more expensive, and many businesses are dropping it. But a Dental $avings Plan might be an affordable benefit that helps out the business owners, their employees and you.

Pitch your savings plan to local businesses. You can even start with business owners who are also patients in your practice. They can offer your plan to their employees and either subsidize it partially or have their employees pay the full cost. They win, because they're offering a new benefit at a time that many of their competitors are cutting back on total compensation. The employees win because even if they have to pay the full cost of plan membership, they get to do it with pre-tax dollars. And finally, you win, because you have a pool of new patients whose benefits are only effective if they receive care at your practice.

I developed my in-house Dental $avings Plan in response to the needs of area senior citizens. However, a plan that provides a good value appeals to everyone, not just Baby Boomers. As you roll out your own savings plan, don't overlook local business owners, and keep an eye out for other underserved groups in your community. When you get new patients into that chair, everyone wins.

You don't have to throw the wine and cheese event model out if you choose to target SMB's. In fact, why not host a similar event for local business owners? You can still sample great wines, snack on yummy cheese and present the benefits of the D$P to a group of folks. Check out the local Chamber of Commerce meeting schedule and offer to host. You can provide breakfast items and coffee if it is a morning meeting or wine and cheese if it is later in the day.

If possible, invite small business owners and their employees at the Chamber to an event at your office. Give them a tour of your office and highlight your unique services, like your Dental $avings Plan that you can offer them. Schedule it at a time that is convenient for them so you increase your chances of a great turnout.

It may be worth setting up a separate small business plan; if a small business guarantees purchase of X plans, you can offer extra services just for them or provide a further price break for the group of plans.

Graduated Care Facilities

While my main focus has been active independent living retirement communities (avoiding assisted living and nursing home facilities) there is another market here you can tap into: graduated care facilities. These facilities typically offer all three types of care for those 55 and older in one location. The key that I found is to find a facility with significantly more active, independent living apartments than assisted or nursing home beds. An example is a facility my mom resides in now, a graduated care facility in South Charlotte, NC. Here they have 150 independent living apartments with around 300 residents. Contrast that with the 30 assisted living and 10 nursing home beds they offer; you can see they have 10x the number of independent living residents as they do assisted living or nursing home care residents. More than enough to warrant a wine and cheese event one time per month until you establish your presence firmly in this community.

Should there be an alternative to wine and cheese?

Thinking about those alternative markets to the independent living community, it also begs the question: What are you offering all the residents in these markets that don't drink wine? Aren't we excluding a good number of our target market sect? Yes, you are! So what kind of event could you offer them instead of wine and cheese? How about an ice cream social? Who doesn't like ice cream? I have fond memories growing up enjoying homemade ice cream and root beer floats with my parents and grandparents. Ice cream socials could be a great way to attract your target market and the patient that may not be into your wine and cheese.

12
HOW TO HOST THE PERFECT EVENT

If dental school didn't teach us much about business, it taught us zero about event planning. In order to help your savings plan promotional event run smoothly, here are a few tips and tricks I have learned to guide you. If you choose to host your own wine and cheese event, connect to whoever is in charge of facility events; oftentimes this is a Facility Director or Special Event Coordinator. Use this checklist to make sure all of your bases have been covered prior to your event. If you appear unprepared at the event, it will reflect poorly on your practice. Let me tell you, no one wants to visit a dentist who seems unprepared or frazzled.

WINE AND CHEESE EVENT CHECKL

DATE:____________ TIME:____________ LOCATION/ROOM: __________

FACILITY CHECKLIST:

- ○ Time and date of event.
- ○ How will people RSVP/ sign up to attend?
- ○ Can you place flyers or signage on campus marketing the event?
- ○ Location of the meeting space on the facility map.
- ○ What time can you arrive to begin set-up?
- ○ What time must you be out of the room?
- ○ Number of tables and chairs
- ○ Room set up (classroom style or round table)
- ○ Is there AV equipment or do you bring your own?
- ○ Is there a screen available?
- ○ Can liquor be served on the premises?
- ○ Are table linens, silverware, plates and glasses provided?
- ○ Are you responsible for clean-up and tear down of tables/chairs etc.?

INTERNAL CHECKLIST:

- ○ How will people sign up for your plan at the event? Do you have a card reader and iPad or will you have them fill out a form?
- ○ Do you need to have materials printed and on hand?
- ○ Will you be offering any give-aways during the event?
- ○ If you are offering a give away, how will people enter to win?
- ○ Will you need pens and paper for attendees to take notes?
- ○ Who will introduce you?
- ○ What will you wear?
- ○ What team members (at least 2) will join the event?
- ○ What will the team member's role be at the event?
- ○ What will the team members wear?
- ○ What will you do if the AV equipment does not work? What is your plan B?
- ○ Will you have a registration limit, both on the high end and low end?
- ○ How many people will need to RSVP in order to confirm the event?
- ○ What is the registration limit in order to have seats for everyone?
- ○ How will attendees contact the office after the event?
- ○ Who will purchase/bring the wine?
- ○ Who will purchase/bring the cheese?
- ○ Who will purchase/bring the plates, cups and napkins?
- ○ Who will bring the wine opener(s)?

is advisable to do a site visit, prior to your event. Ask to see the space and get a sense for how you want the event to feel. For example, if round tables are available, think about advantages and disadvantages to such a seating arrangement. Will you ask people to turn their chairs to face you? Or, will you walk amongst the tables so everyone can see and hear you without moving their seats? Is your presentation interactive? Do participants need a writing surface if they would like to sign up for your Dental $avings Plan at the event? The more prepared you can be for your event; the more smoothly it will go. You don't want to appear unprepared, nervous or thrown off by things you could have been prepared for.

A few words of advice

We have learned many lessons along the way. I want to make sure you are privy to all of them, so you can have a smoother ride than I did.

What to wear

Wear your lab coat, period. These people are coming to see an expert, so it is important to look the part. In my experience and my research on influence, tapping into the power of Authority by looking the part of an authoritative figure will pay off. Attendees will also be able to spot you easily in the crowd if they have questions for the doctor.

Which team members should join?

I always bring at least two team members. They are responsible for serving the wine and cheese as well as greeting attendees as they arrive. I always bring my Treatment Coordinator, the person in charge of processing payments. My team members are positive, outgoing and engaging—providing the perfect image of our office to attendees.

What kind of wine is best?

I love to tell attendees, "If you can't get to Napa, we'll bring Napa Valley to you!" Since tastes vary so greatly, I prefer to bring an assortment. For reds, I will bring a few bottles of Pinot Noir and Cabernet Sauvignon. For white, I stick to Pinot Grigio and Chardonnay. I like to bring wines from the Napa Valley, but you don't have to. I do suggest bringing a more expensive bottle to pour first. It is important to have an alternative to wine. Bring some chilled bottles of water or seltzer.

What about the cheese?

One lesson we learned early on is people eat way less than you expect. Typically for an event we bring one cheese and fruit platter, and it is plenty. You can choose to serve some crackers or nuts as well, but don't feel like you need to feed the crowd an entire meal. Most of the time we go home with extra food, and it is a waste. When in doubt, bring more wine.

Who should introduce you?

While it may seem funny at first, it is best to have someone else introduce you to your audience. In the beginning, I had a team member begin the evening with a short bio and introduction. Again, this reinforces your Authority and gives the audience a chance to learn a bit about you. Now that we have patients in these communities, I will often ask one of them to give a short introduction and testimony about their experience. This also builds upon your Authority, as the testimonial can speak to your trustworthiness. Furthermore, attach it to the Principle of Liking as the audience sees someone just like them, who lives in this community and chooses you. I have found this to be wildly successful and the patient is typically thrilled to speak about their experience. Below is a sample of an introduction one of my patients gives for me.

Introduction for Dr. Phelps' Sun City Wine and Cheese Events

"Hi, my name is Jesse Samples, current resident here at Sun City and a patient of Dr. Phelps for a while now. Just to tell you a little about Dr. Phelps—He was born and raised in Greensboro, North Carolina. After obtaining his bachelor's degree from the University of North Carolina at Chapel Hill, he earned his dental degree Nova Southeastern University in Ft. Lauderdale, Florida. You all need to believe him when he says they aren't like most dental offices. The entire staff treats you like family and really listens to your dental concerns. I grew up in times of hardship and through the war; I did not take great care of my teeth, so I needed a lot of attention to my oral health. Finally, I found my dental home when I met Dr. Phelps and his staff. If it wasn't for their CT scan, I could have been in major trouble! The scan showed Dr. Phelps where my sinuses fell, which helped him know where he could place an implant without damaging my sinuses. If I ever have any dental issues, all I have to do is call and they work with me to find a convenient time. When Dr. Phelps is not available, he has trained the other doctors in the same philosophies and will take great care of you too. Looking for a top of the notch dental team, you cannot go wrong with Dr. Phelps and his staff!"

What should the presentation include?

It is tempting to make the presentation all about the

Dental $avings Plan; after all, that is what you are there to sell. However, these folks don't want to sit through a sales pitch, even if there is great wine. Here is my general format:

1. Short introduction to my office

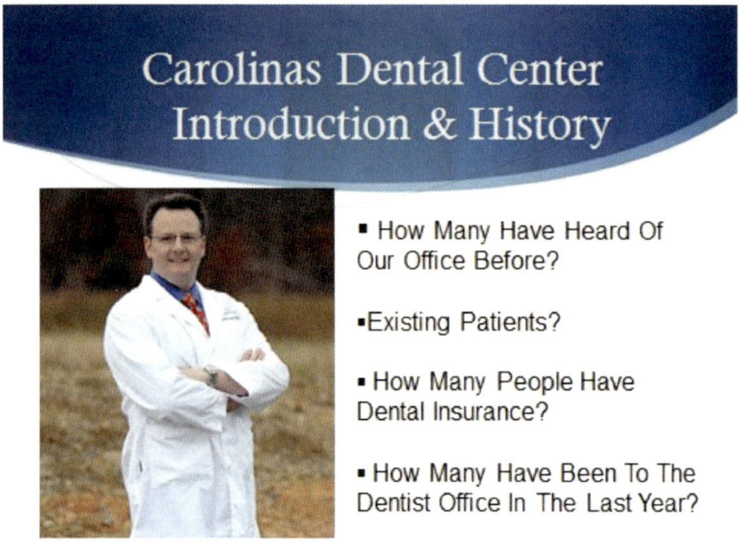
Carolinas Dental Center
Introduction & History
▪ How Many Have Heard Of Our Office Before?
▪Existing Patients?
▪ How Many People Have Dental Insurance?
▪ How Many Have Been To The Dentist Office In The Last Year?

2. Short introduction of my family

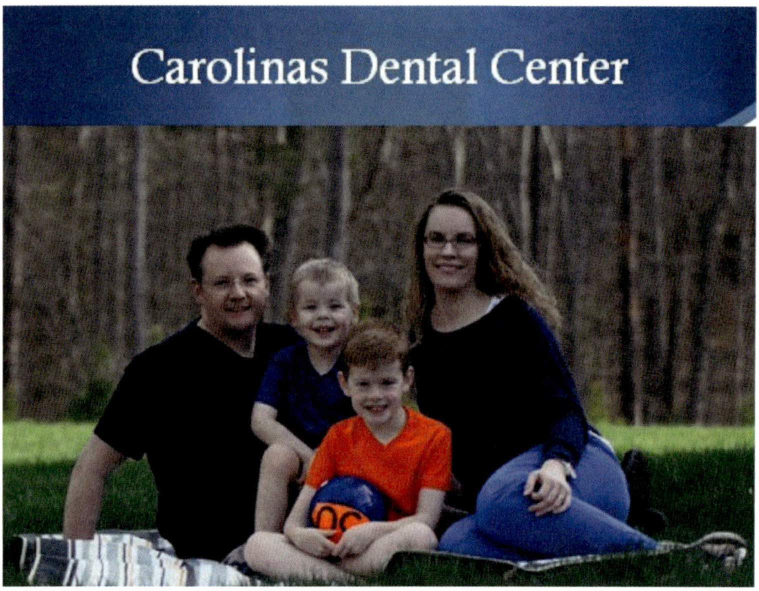
Carolinas Dental Center

3. Short introduction of the team

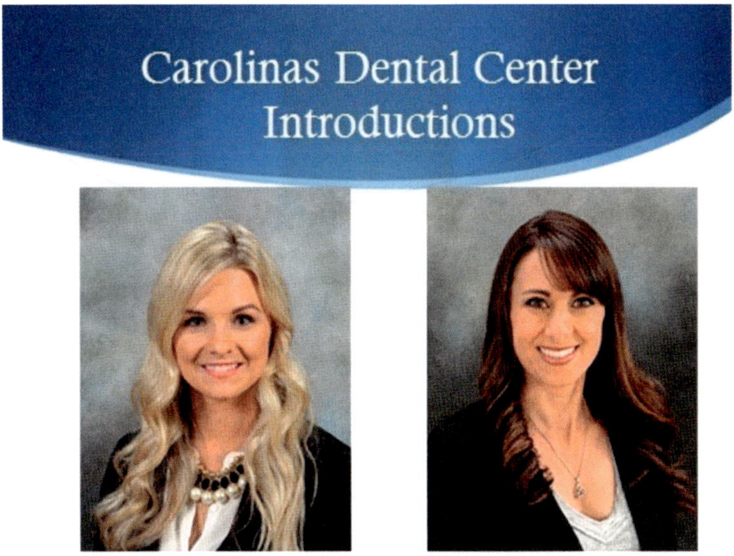

4. Map of their location with the route to your office highlighted.

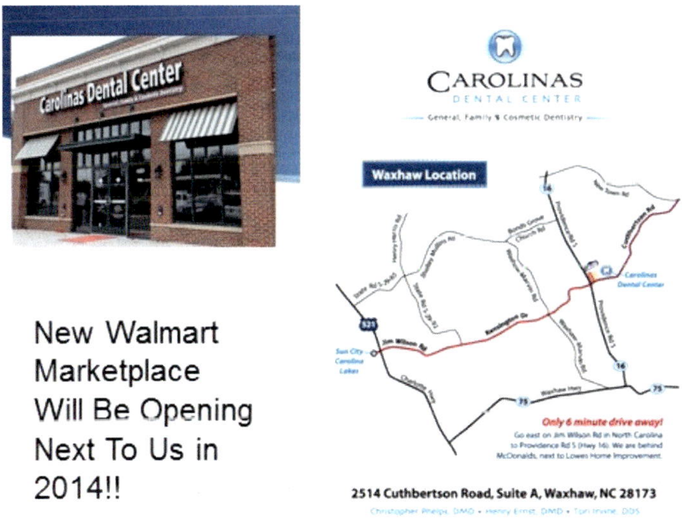

5. Overview of how my office is different from other offices in the area whose advertising they may have seen.

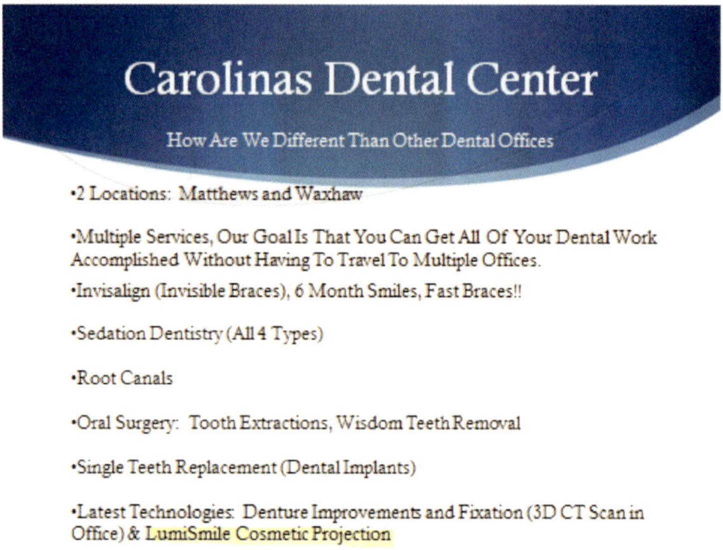

6. Focus on how I treat their specific needs like sedation dentistry, alternative office hours and the Dental $avings Plan.

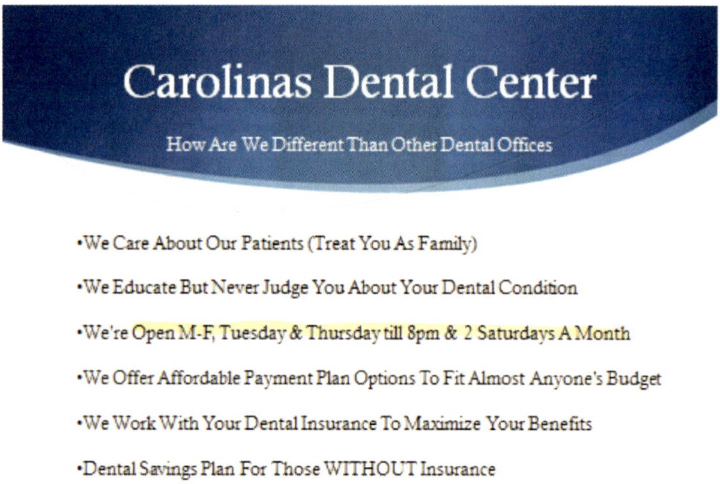

7. Provide educational information

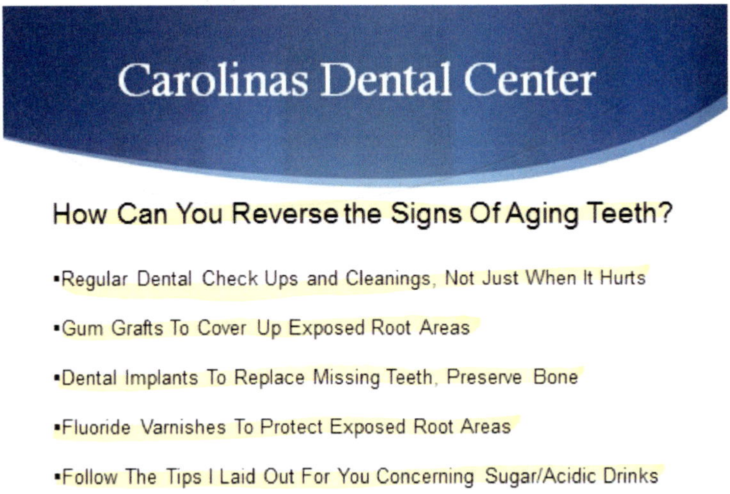

Your presentation should keep moving. Don't bore the audience to death with complicated dental terminology; make it interesting and relevant to them. They should leave the presentation feeing educated, not sold to.

How to elevate your event

If you do multiple events and decide you want to step it up, giveaways are an excellent way to add excitement. We regularly offer giveaways, and it has been wildly successful. The seniors love it and it provides an opportunity to show how much we care for the community.

Raffles are an easy way to get everyone involved and engaged through the end of the presentation. We hand out raffle tickets during the presentation and draw winners at the end. Prizes vary; everything from portable sports folding chairs to a free Dental $avings Plan. I give away a certificate for a free one-hour tooth whitening ($575 value) or it can be used as in-office credit for any procedure over $1000. I have also experimented with larger giveaways and had great success.

Larger giveaways can do two things for you. It could be the first thing you promote to these communities as a way to get maximum exposure or word of mouth for your first several wine and cheese events. If you have already started doing these events and notice your attendance numbers flatlining they can also help get the community reengaged with your message. After doing the wine and cheese seminars once a month for over a year, I noticed my attendance numbers were topping out at around 50% of what they used to be. Seeing how much they enjoyed the smaller giveaways we raffled off at the end of each event, I began wondering what larger item I could give one of them a chance to win. After surveying many of our existing patients from this community, I discovered they all share the same major expense, homeowners association dues. As I mentioned before, knowing they think they can't afford $600 dental insurance, I am sure they don't like to pay the HOA dues, which can range anywhere from $1800-$2300 per year. From that realization, came my HOA giveaway.

The following month I used my full page ad in the community magazine to promote the contest. For one lucky winner, I would pay their HOA dues in full for the year. There were three major rules to the contest and no purchase was necessary.

1. They had to attend one of my next three wine and cheese events.

Limiting the number of chances to win comes from the Scarcity Principle and is a powerful motivator for action today.

2. They had to drop off their raffle ticket in my office.

While attending a wine and cheese event, they were each given a red raffle ticket. To be entered officially into the contest, all they had to do was come by my dental office and drop it off. They could come in for their cleaning and drop it off, they could come in for a consult with a doctor and drop it off, or they could come in and take a new patient tour and drop it off after. But, they had to come to the office to drop off the ticket to be entered into the contest.

Over the next three months, the attendance at my wine and cheese events exploded. What's more, the new patient numbers in my office went from an average of

30 per month to 69 per month. At the end of the three months, I decided to throw a big party to announce the winner. I ended up with 90 people submitting their tickets. This led to rule three.

3. You had to be present at the giveaway party when the winner was announced.

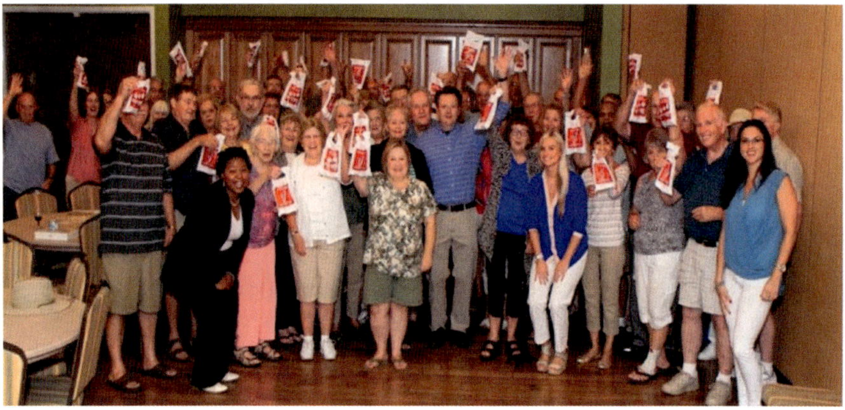

Attendees at the HOA giveaway event

For the winner, I paid $2200 for her HOA dues. To reciprocate, she referred four patients to my office and had five crowns done. On top of this, I used the Principle of Consistency to influence all 90 attendees to refer 90 more patients to the practice. So I ask you, did it really cost me anything?

The key to the success of your program is to be creative and talk to your market. What do they want? Where are they spending money that is a hassle?

Where can you step in and give them a chance to wi something meaningful?

Of course, you have all the tools you could possibly need to replicate my 1.4 million dollar success right here in this book. But if you are like most that are short on time and motivation to start this by yourself, check out www.MembershipSavingsPlan.com and let our team help!

13
YOU CAN DO THIS

Private practice doctors are a tenacious lot. We have grit, guts and more willpower than most to get the job done. We all spend too much time spinning our wheels with marketing efforts that just don't work. In this book, I have shown how I found a way to market directly to people who were *actively seeking dental care.* In my case, this was retirees. I went directly to their communities and combined talks on dental health with wine and cheese socials. This gave me a chance to approach a friendly audience with targeted information and advice. As a result, I could attract 60 new patients a month for less than the cost of a tiny newspaper advertisement in a local paper.

You may be trying to attract families with children, young professionals or local employers to your practice, but the theory behind the wine and cheese socials remains the same. Meet your potential patients where they are, make meeting with you a treat, and explain what your practice has to offer them at their stage in life. Spend your marketing dollars on people who are looking for a dentist in your area, not whoever happens to be listening to the radio at 5 am on a Saturday morning. Get creative, and be specific. You'll see greater returns on your marketing dollars and give your practice a chance to grow.

On top of that, I've found the Dental $avings Plan is the best way to attract new fee-for-service patients to your practice. Patients love to know that they're saving money on high-quality dental care, and seniors living on fixed incomes appreciate the predictability that comes with a Dental $avings Plan. As a business owner, there is nothing better than a prime market, the perfect message and a medium that involves wine and cheese to seal the deal for me. I truly hope my 1.4 million dollars of growth in just 24 months (with all the lessons I learned along the way) is motivating. I hope the tools and tips in this book solidify your resolve to make a Dental $avings Plan work for your office. It can, and it will, with a little hard work and maybe just a little wine.

Cheers to your success!

Dr. Christopher Phelps DMD.

About the Author

Dr. Phelps is a general dentist who was born and raised in Greensboro, North Carolina. He moved to Charlotte in 2003 with his wife Amber and enjoys playing tennis and spending time with his two boys, Riley and Liam. After obtaining his bachelor's degree from the University of North Carolina at Chapel Hill, he earned his dental degree magnum cum laude from the prestigious Nova Southeastern University College of Dental Medicine in Ft. Lauderdale, Florida where he was awarded awards from the Academy of General Dentistry for "Excellence in General Dentistry" and was inducted into the Omicron Kappa Upsilon National Dental Honor Society, which only admits the top 5% of each graduating dental class throughout the country.

Dr. Phelps has had the pleasure of providing the cosmetic dentistry for "Charlotte's Complete Makeover," an extreme makeover contest held in conjunction with Dr. Victor Ferrari, plastic surgeon, and Dr. Jonathan Christenbury, LASIKTM eye surgeon. In addition, Dr. Phelps has had several of his articles published in peer-reviewed dental journals concerning cosmetic and implant dentistry. Dr. Phelps strives to be on the leading edge of dentistry but not the bleeding edge, ultimately providing his patients with all the latest available technologies and options for their optimum dental health.

Dr. Phelps is a member of the American Dental Association, North Carolina Dental Society, American Academy of Cosmetic Dentistry, and Academy of General Dentistry. He has received certification in sedation dentistry from the Dental Organization for Conscious Sedation (D.O.C.S.) and has been awarded one of Charlotte's Best Dentists numerous times over the last 10 years. In addition, he was given the Doctor's Choice Award in March of 2016, which was voted on solely by other dentists and physicians. In September of 2016, he was named as one of the top 100 doctors throughout the US.

Dr. Phelps spends his time in the practice focused on Sedation Dentistry and Dental Implant cases. His other passion is mentoring, coaching and training other General Dentists through The Phelps Institute. The Institute offers a slew of trainings including a 2-day marketing workshop to attract a better quality patient. Attendees learn how to apply Dr. Cialdini's 6 Principles of Persuasion and Ethical Influence in office. In addition the Phelps Institute is one of the few locations in the entire US that trains General Dentists, from any state, how to surgically place dental implants on live patients (not models or cadavers). Check out these and other trainings at www.DrPhelpsHelps.com or www.ThePhelpsInstitute.com

www.MembershipSavingsPlan.com

Acknowledgments

Someone wise once said, "Never stop learning because life never stops teaching." After 18 years of marriage, watching my two boys grow up and over 13 years of clinical practice I can honestly say, truer words have never been spoken. Because of the path I've been on, I have learned so many valuable lessons over the years from so many people, but my colleagues and patients have been some of the most important. From my talks with my patients, they have inspired me with new marketing ideas and mediums to get my messages out there to more just like them. By listening and interacting with them, I learn how to identify new barriers that are keeping more patients from coming into my practice. This is valuable insight which teaches me how to create new solutions to help them get around these barriers.

For over 9 years, I've had the honor of educating and training my fellow colleagues. Your dedication to improving the practice of dentistry is inspiring to say the least. Our time together has taught me the obstacles you've faced with getting more new patients in the door, setting the stage for more of them to say yes to your treatment recommendations, and how to add more services to your practice to help you succeed today and survive tomorrow's tough dental economy. It's because of these continued obstacles we all face in practice that I'm pleased to announce the launch of The Phelps Institute. A new series of training programs that cover every aspect of our dental practice and help you take these concepts to solving your practices issues and helping you turn them into practice. These are tried and true workshops and continuums that I've developed that have been successful for my practices as well as those of dentists all over the country. I invite you to join me and my team at The Phelps Institute in Charlotte North Carolina, and I'll even make sure you enjoy a nice glass of wine while we continue to learn and teach each other.

Thanks for reading! Please add a short review on Amazon and let me know what you thought!

References

i When You Need A Dentist. (n.d.). Retrieved May 17, 2016, from www.superteeth.com

ii The Business of Oral Health Care: A Look Into the Corporatization of American Dentistry. (n.d.). Retrieved May 17, 2016, from www.lmtmag.com/articles/ the_business_of_oral_health_care_a_look_into_the_corporatization_of_american_dentistry

iii ADA Explores Growth of Large Group Practices. (2012, April 9). Retrieved May 17, 2016, from www.ada.org/ en/publications/ada-news/2012-archive/april/ada-explores-growth-of-large-group-practices

iv Private equity investment in healthcare: 15 healthcare investment niches — A review of key sectors for 2015. (n.d.). Retrieved May 17, 2016, from www.beckershospitalreview.com/finance/private-equity-investment-in-healthcare-15-healthcare-investment- niches-a-review-of-key-sectors-for-2015.html

v 8 of the Most Interesting things we are seeing in Healthcare. (n.d.). Retrieved May 17, 2016, from www.beckershospitalreview.com/white-papers/8-of-the-most-interesting-things-we-are-seeing-in- healthcare.html

vi Dental Benefits Basics - Who. (n.d.). Retrieved May 17, 2016, from www.nadp.org/ Dental_Benefits_Basics/Dental_BB_1.aspx

vii What is the Value of a New Dental Patient? (n.d.). Re- trieved May 18, 2016, from www.wpicommunications.com/ articles/what-is-the-value-of- a-new-dental-patient/

viii DELG Survey. (2014, November). Retrieved May 18, 2016, from www.levingroup.com/pdf/ DELGSurvey_Article_Nov2014.pdf

ix (n.d.). Retrieved May 18, 2016, from www.adweek.com/

x Social Demographic Differences - News, Habits & At- titudes. (n.d.). Retrieved May 21, 2016, from www.americanpressinstitute.org/publications/reports/ survey-research/social-demographic-differences-news- habits-attitudes/

xi (n.d.). Retrieved May 19, 2016, from www.ada.org/~/media/ADA/MemberCenter/FIles/Escan2013_Diringer_Full.

xii Olenski, S. (2015, June 5). 7 Reasons Why Marketing to Baby Boomers is Unique. Retrieved May 19, 2016, from www.forbes.com/sites/steveolenski/2015/06/05/7-reasons-why-marketing-to-baby-boomers-is-unique/ #32a1e4ef73de

xiii 50 Facts and Fiction: Size, Wealth and Spending of 50 Consumers. (n.d.). Retrieved May 19, 2016, from www.immersionactive.com/resources/size-wealth-spending -50-consumers/

xiv The Hottest Trends in Boomer Travel. (2013, August 1). Retrieved May 19, 2016, from www.forbes.com/ sites/nextavenue/2013/08/01/the-hottest-trends-in-boomer -travel/#54360abb2cd4

xv For Advertisers, Baby Boomers Are A Market Hiding In Plain Sight. (n.d.). Retrieved May 19, 2016, from www.npr.org/2015/05/02/403766871/for-advertisers-baby-boom ers-are-a-market-hiding-in-plain-sight

xvi Cosmetic Dentistry - The Boom is Upon Us. (n.d.). Re- trieved May 19, 2016, from www.dentaleconomics.com/articles/print/volume-91/ issue-9/features/cosmetic-dentistry-the-boom-is-upon- us.html

xvii (n.d.). Retrieved May 19, 2016, from www.ada.org/~/media/ADA/MemberCenter /FIles/Escan2013_Diringer_Full.ashx)

xviii How Millennials Are Changing the Face of Marketing Forever. (n.d.). Retrieved May 22, 2016, from www.bcgperspectives.com/content/articles/market- ing_center_c onsumer_customer_insight_how_millennials_changing_marketing_forever/?chapte r=3

xix How to develop an Ideal Patient Profile to attract the right patients to your practice. (n.d.). Retrieved May 22, 2016, from www.reminmedia.com/how-to-develop-an- ideal-patient-profile-to-attract-the-right-patients-to- your-practice/

xx Hogshead, S. (n.d.). Fascinate: Your 7 Triggers to Per- suasion and Captivation. Retrieved May 22, 2016, from www.amazon.com/Fascinate-Your-Triggers- Persuasion -Captivation/dp/0061714704/ref=sr_1_2? s=books&ie=UTF8&qid=1463938843&sr=1-2&keywords=facinate

xxi 4 Ways to Market to Baby Boomers. (2015). Retrieved May 21, 2016, from www.magicblog.magiconline.com/ content/4-ways-to-market-baby-boomers-2015

xxii Number of Millennial Wine Drinkers Catches Boomers (n.d.). Retrieved May 21, 2016 from http://www.winesandvines.com/template.cfm? section=news&content=166 313

xxiii AARP Dental Insurance Plan. (n.d.). Retrieved June 2, 2016, from www.delta dentalins.com/aarp/index.html

xxiv Amazon Prime: Bigger, More Powerful, More Profitable Than Anyone Imagined. (2013, March 18). Retrieved June 2, 2016, from www.business.time.com/ 2013/03/18/amazon- prime-bigger-more-powerful-more-profitable-than-anyone-imagined/

xxv Know the Rules before Rewarding Patients for Referrals. (n.d.). Retrieved June 2, 2016, from www.fluenceportland.com/strategy/know-the-rules-before-rewar ding-patients-for-referrals

xxvi Cialdini, R. B., PhD. (n.d.). Influence: The Power of Persuasion. Retrieved June 2, 2016, from www.amazon.com/Influence-Psychology-Persuasion- Robert-Cial dini/dp/006124189X

xxvii Demographic Maps: Aging (n.d.). Retrieved August 17, 2016, from www.north carolinahealthnews.org/2015/06/30/making-the- case-for-aing-in-place/

Made in the USA
San Bernardino, CA
20 November 2019

60205047R00062